ıne World Health Report 2013

Research for Universal Health Coverage

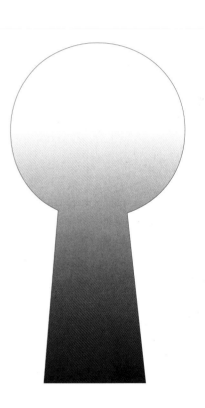

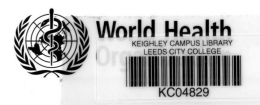

World Health

WHO Library Cataloguing-in-Publication Data

The world health report 2013: research for universal health coverage.

1.World health - trends. 2.Universal coverage. 3.Health services accessibility. 4.Research. 5.Insurance, Health.
I.World Health Organization.

ISBN 978 92 4 156459 5   (NLM classification: W 84.6)
ISBN 978 92 4 069081 3 (ePub)
ISBN 978 92 4 069082 0 (Daisy)
ISBN 978 92 4 069083 7 (PDF)
ISSN 1020-3311

Acknowledgements

Under the aegis of Assistant Directors-General Hiroki Nakatani and Marie-Paule Kieny, the following people wrote and produced this report:

Lead authors

Christopher Dye, Ties Boerma, David Evans, Anthony Harries, Christian Lienhardt, Joanne McManus, Tikki Pang, Robert Terry, Rony Zachariah.

WHO staff in Geneva

Caroline Allsopp, Najeeb Al-Shorbaji, John Beard, Douglas Bettcher, Diarmid Campbell-Lendrum, Andrew Cassels, A'Isha Commar, Luis De Francisco Serpa, Carlos Dora, Gerald Dziekan, Christy Feig, Fiona Fleck, Haileyesus Getahun, Abdul Ghaffar, Laragh Gollogly, Andre Griekspoor, Sophie Guetaneh Aguettant, Metin Gülmezoglu, Ali Hamandi, Asli Kalin, Ghassan Karam, Edward Kelley, Richard Laing, Melanie Lauckner, Knut Lönroth, Mary MacLennan, Clarisse Mason, Elizabeth Mason, Mike Mbizvo, Shanti Mendis, Thierry Mertens, Zafar Mirza, Maria Neira, Ulysses Panisset, Kimberly Parker, Michaela Pfeiffer, Kent Ranson, Mario Raviglione, John Reeder, Alex Ross, Cathy Roth, Sarah Russell, Ritu Sadana, Abha Saxena, Trish Saywell, Thomas Shakespeare, Isobel Sleeman, Johannes Sommerfeld, Marleen Temmerman, Diana Weil, Karin Weyer.

WHO staff in regional and country offices

Naeema Al-Gasseer, Luis Cuervo Amore, Govin Permanand, Manju Rani, Issa Sanou, Gunawan Setiadi, Claudia Stein, Edouard Tursan d'Espaignet, Adik Wibowo.

Members of the Scientific Advisory Panel

Andy Haines (chair), Fred Binka, Somsak Chunharas, Maimunah Hamid, Richard Horton, John Lavis, Hassan Mshinda, Pierre Ongolo-Zogo, Silvina Ramos, Francisco Songane.

Other individuals who contributed to or reviewed the content

Claire Allen, Thomas Bombelles, David Bramley, Martin Buxton, Anne Candau, Michael Clarke, Sylvia de Haan, David Durrheim, Toker Ergüder, Mahmoud Fathalla, Stephen Hanney, Mark Harrington, Sue Hobbs, Carel IJsselmuiden, Nasreen Jessani, Anatole Krattiger, Gina Lagomarsino, Guillermo Lemarchand, David Mabey, Dermot Maher, Cristina Ortiz, Adolfo Martinez Palomo, Charlotte Masiello-Riome, Peter Massey, Martin Mckee, Opena Merlita, Amanda Milligan, Peter Ndumbe, Thomson Prentice, Bernd Rechel, Jan Ross, Sabine Schott, Peter Small, Hanna Steinbach, Sheri Strite, Yot Teerawattananon, Göran Tomson, Ian Viney, Laetitia Voneche, Shaw Voon Wong, Judith Whitworth, Suwit Wibulpolprasert, Catherine Wintrich.

"Universal health coverage is the single most powerful concept that public health has to offer"

Dr Margaret Chan, Address to the Sixty-fifth
World Health Assembly, May 2012

"Another lesson is the importance of long-term investment in the research institutions that generate evidence for policy ..."

Lancet, 2012, 380:1259,
on the approach to universal health coverage in Mexico

Message from the Director-General

As we approach the 2015 deadline for meeting the United Nations Millennium Development Goals (MDGs), it is time to take stock of the progress that has been made since 2000. It is also time to reflect on how we made progress, and on how we could do better.

All eight of the MDGs have consequences for health, but three put health at front and centre – they concern child health (MDG 4), maternal health (MDG 5), and the control of HIV/AIDS, malaria, tuberculosis and other major communicable diseases (MDG 6). To highlight just one of these, MDG 4 calls for a reduction in the number of child deaths from 12 million in 1990 to fewer than 4 million by 2015. Although great strides have been taken since the turn of the millennium, especially in reducing deaths after the neonatal period, the best measurements indicate that nearly 7 mil-

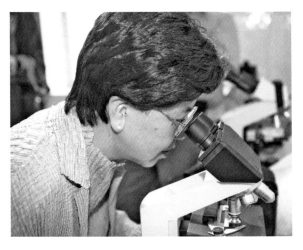

lion children under five years of age died in 2011. From experience in high-income countries, we know that almost all of these deaths can be prevented. But how can that be done everywhere?

One idea is to make greater use of community-based interventions. But do they work? Experiments in the form of randomized controlled trials provide the most persuasive evidence for action in public health. By 2010, 18 such trials in Africa, Asia and Europe had shown that the participation of outreach workers, lay health workers, community midwives, community and village health workers, and trained birth attendants collectively reduced neonatal deaths by an average of 24%, stillbirths by 16% and perinatal mortality by 20%. Maternal illness was also reduced by a quarter (1). These

1. Lassi ZS, Haider BA, Bhutta ZA. Community-based intervention packages for reducing maternal and neonatal morbidity and mortality and improving neonatal outcomes. *Cochrane Database of Systematic Reviews (Online)*, 2010,11:CD007754. PMID:21069697

trials clearly do not give all the answers – for instance, the benefits of these interventions in reducing maternal mortality, as distinct from morbidity, are still unclear – but they are a powerful argument for involving community health workers in the care of mothers and newborn children.

These rigorous investigations have the potential to benefit millions around the world. They confront the challenge presented by just one of the MDGs, but they capture the general spirit of this report – to promote investigations in which creativity is harnessed by the highest-quality science in order to deliver affordable, quality health services and better health for everyone. More than that, the process of discovery is a source of inspiration and motivation, stirring ambitions to defeat the biggest problems in public health. This is the purpose of *Research for universal health coverage*.

This report is for everyone concerned with understanding how to reach the goal of universal health coverage – those who fund the necessary research, those who do research and who would like to do research, and those who use the evidence from research. It shows how research for health in general underpins research for universal health coverage in particular.

Understanding how to make progress towards achieving the MDGs is central to this report. But its scope is wider. As the 2015 deadline draws closer, we are looking for ways to improve all aspects of health, working within and beyond the MDG framework. And we are investigating how better health can contribute to the larger goal of human development. In this broad context, I invite you to read *Research for universal health coverage*. I invite you to assess the report's arguments, review its evidence, and help support the research that will bring us closer to the goal of universal health coverage.

Dr Margaret Chan
Director-General
World Health Organization

Contents

Executive summary

Three key messages from *The world health report*

- Universal health coverage, with full access to high-quality services for health promotion, prevention, treatment, rehabilitation, palliation and financial risk protection, cannot be achieved without evidence from research. Research has the power to address a wide range of questions about how we can reach universal coverage, providing answers to improve human health, well-being and development.
- All nations should be producers of research as well as consumers. The creativity and skills of researchers should be used to strengthen investigations not only in academic centres but also in public health programmes, close to the supply of and demand for health services.
- Research for universal health coverage requires national and international backing. To make the best use of limited resources, systems are needed to develop national research agendas, to raise funds, to strengthen research capacity, and to make appropriate and effective use of research findings.

Why universal health coverage?

In 2005, all WHO Member States made the commitment to achieve universal health coverage. The commitment was a collective expression of the belief that all people should have access to the health services they need without risk of financial ruin or impoverishment. Working towards universal health coverage is a powerful mechanism for achieving better health and well-being, and for promoting human development.

Chapter 1 explains how the resolution adopted by all WHO Member States embraces the two facets of universal health coverage: the provision of, and access to, high-quality health services; and financial risk protection for people who need to use these services. "Health services" in this report mean methods for promotion, prevention, treatment, rehabilitation and palliation, encompassing health care in communities, health centres and hospitals. The term includes ways of taking action on social and environmental determinants both within and beyond the health sector. Financial risk protection is part of the package of measures that provides overall social protection.

Why research?

Scientific research has been fundamental to the improvement of human health. Research is vital in developing the technology, systems and services needed to achieve universal health coverage. On the road to universal coverage, taking a methodical approach to formulating and answering questions is not a luxury but a necessity.

When WHO Member States made the pledge to achieve universal coverage they took a significant step forward for public health. As described in **Chapter 1**, taking that step effectively launched an agenda for research. In this report, research is the set of formal methods that turns promising ideas into practical solutions for improving health services, and consequently for improving health. The goal of the report is to identify the research questions that open the way to universal health coverage and to discuss how these questions can be answered.

Many recent advances have been made in health service coverage and in financial risk protection as shown, for example, by progress towards the United Nations Millennium Development Goals (MDGs). Despite this progress, the gap between the present coverage of health services and universal health coverage remains large for many conditions of ill-health in many settings. For instance, nearly half of all HIV-infected people eligible for antiretroviral therapy were still not receiving it in 2011, and an estimated 150 million people suffer financial catastrophe each year because they have to pay cash out-of-pocket for the health care they need. The focus of this report is on the research needed to provide wider access to essential services of this kind, and how to create the environment in which this research can be carried out.

What questions need to be answered by research?

Chapter 1 identifies research questions of two kinds. The causes of ill-health differ from one setting to another and so too must the necessary health services, including mechanisms for financial risk protection. The first group of questions therefore asks how to choose the health services needed in each setting, how to improve service coverage and financial protection, and consequently how to protect and improve health and well-being.

These questions throw up a wide range of topics for research. Research is needed to find out how to improve the coverage of existing interventions and how to select and introduce new ones. Research must explore the development and use of both "software" (such as schemes for financial protection and simplified approaches to treatment) and "hardware" (research and development for commodities and technology). And research is needed to investigate ways of improving health from within and outside the health sector.

The most pressing research questions have been identified for many specific health topics, such as maternal and child health, communicable diseases, and health systems and services. Although there are notable exceptions, less effort has generally been given worldwide to establishing and publicizing national research priorities, to assessing the strengths and weaknesses of national research programmes, and to evaluating the health, social and economic benefits of research.

The second group of questions asks how to measure progress towards universal coverage in each setting for each population, in terms of the services that are needed and the indicators and data that measure the coverage of these services. The answer to this group of questions is a measure of the gap between the present coverage of services and universal coverage. The challenge for research is to fill that gap.

Many specific indicators, targets and data sources are already used to measure the coverage of specific health interventions. The metrics used to monitor progress towards the MDGs track, for example, access to antiretroviral therapy, births attended by skilled health personnel, and immunization coverage. However, the measurement of other aspects of coverage needs further development; interventions to prevent and control noncommunicable diseases, or to track healthy ageing, are two examples.

It is not usually possible to measure the coverage of the hundreds of interventions and services that make up a national health system. However, it is possible to choose a subset of services, with their associated indicators, that are representative of the overall quantity, quality, equity and financing of services. Then a practical definition of universal health coverage is that all persons who are eligible have access to the services they need. To choose the essential health services that should be monitored, and a set of indicators to track progress towards universal coverage, is a research task for health programmes in each country. Out of these investigations will emerge a common set of indicators that can be used to measure and compare progress towards universal health coverage across all countries.

With its focus on research, the goal of this report is not to measure definitively the gap between the present coverage of health services and universal coverage but, instead, to identify the questions that arise as we move towards universal coverage and to discuss how these questions can be answered.

Should all countries have the capacity to do research?

The results of some research studies are widely applicable, but many questions about universal health coverage require local answers. All countries therefore need to be producers of research as well as consumers of it. An abundance of data, presented in **Chapter 2**, shows that most low- and middle-income countries now have, at least, the foundations on which to build effective national health research systems. Some countries have much more than the foundations; they have thriving research communities with a growing number of "south–south" as well as "north–south" international links. By strengthening these systems, countries will be able to capitalize more effectively on the supply of ideas, using formal research methods to turn them into useful products and strategies for better health.

Which kinds of research studies have shown how to improve the coverage of health services and how to improve health?

The case for investing in research is made, in part, by demonstrating that scientific investigations really do produce results that can be translated into accessible and affordable health services that provide benefits for health. **Chapter 3** presents 12 examples of studies that show how research can address some of the major questions about achieving universal health coverage, and can deliver results that have influenced, or could influence, policy and health outcomes.

Three examples make the point. In one, a systematic review of survey data from 22 African countries showed how the use of insecticide-treated mosquito nets was associated with fewer malaria infections and lower mortality in young children. This evidence underlines the value of scaling up and maintaining coverage of insecticide-treated nets in malaria-endemic areas. In a second set of experimental trials in Ethiopia, Kenya, Sudan and Uganda, a combination of the drugs sodium stibogluconate and paromomycin was found to be an effective treatment for visceral leishmaniasis. Treatment with the drug combination is shorter than with sodium stibogluconate alone and is less likely to lead to drug resistance. On the basis of these findings, WHO recommended the drug combination as a first-line treatment for visceral leishmaniasis in East Africa. A third systematic review of evidence from Brazil, Colombia, Honduras, Malawi, Mexico and Nicaragua showed how conditional cash transfers – cash payments made in return for using health services – encourage the use of these services and lead to better health outcomes.

The successes of these investigations, and the others described in **Chapter 3**, should be a stimulus to invest in further research. Not all investigations will find that ideas for improving health services are successful, or that the provision of new services actually improves health. In mapping the route to universal coverage, the negative results of research studies are just as valuable as the positive ones.

Which research methods are used to answer questions about universal health coverage?

The examples described in **Chapter 3** expose the diversity of questions about universal health coverage, and also the variety of research methods used to investigate them. Methods include quantitative and qualitative evaluations, observational and case-control studies, intervention studies, randomized controlled trials, and systematic reviews and meta-analyses. The report shows the benefits of having evidence from multiple sources, explores the link between experimental design and strength of inference, and highlights the compromises in study design (better evidence is often more costly, but not always) that must be made by all investigators. The survey of research methods reveals the nature of the research cycle, where questions lead to answers that lead to yet more questions. The chapter illustrates some of the ways in which research is linked with health policy and practice.

What can be done to strengthen national health research systems?

Research is likely to be most productive when it is conducted within a supportive national research system. **Chapter 4** is an introduction to the essential functions of national health research systems, namely: to set research priorities, to develop research capacity, to define norms and standards for research, and to translate evidence into practice.

Standard methods have been developed to set research priorities. These methods should be used more widely by governments to set national priorities across all aspects of health and to determine how best to spend limited funds on research.

With regard to strengthening capacity, effective research needs transparent and accountable methods for allocating funds, in addition to well-equipped research institutions and networks. However, it is the people who do research – with their curiosity, imagination, motivation, technical skills, experience and connections – that are most critical to the success of the research enterprise.

Codes of practice, which are the cornerstone of any research system, are already in use in many countries. The task ahead is to ensure that such codes of practice are comprehensive and apply in all countries, and to encourage adherence everywhere.

Achieving universal health coverage depends on research ranging from studies of causation to studies of how health systems function. However, because many existing cost-effective interventions are not widely used, there is a particular need to close the gap between existing knowledge and action. Areas of research that need special attention concern the implementation of new and existing technologies, health service operations, and the design of effective health systems. To help bridge the gap between science and practice, research should be strengthened not only in academic centres but also in public health programmes, close to the supply of and demand for health services.

How can research for universal health coverage be supported nationally and internationally?

In the wake of many previous reports, **Chapter 4** presents three mechanisms to stimulate and facilitate research for universal health coverage – monitoring, coordination and financing. Provided there is a commitment to share data, national and global observatories could be established to monitor research activities. Observatories could serve a variety of functions, acting as repositories of data on the process of doing research and presenting and sharing the findings of research studies. Such data would help in tracking progress towards universal health coverage, country by country.

Monitoring supports the second function, coordination, on various levels – by sharing information, by jointly setting research priorities, or by facilitating collaboration on research projects.

Regarding the third function, financing, health research is more effective and productive if there is a guaranteed, regular income. Sustained financing guarantees that research projects are not interrupted or otherwise compromised by a sudden lack of resources. Various mechanisms for raising and disbursing additional research funds have been proposed and are under discussion. Whatever mechanism is adopted, international donors and national governments should measure progress against their own commitments to investing in health research.

How will WHO support research for universal health coverage?

Chapter 5 draws out the dominant themes of the report, and proposes a set of actions by which the research community, national governments, donors, civil society and international organizations, including WHO, can support the research that is needed if we are to reach universal health coverage.

Although the debate about universal health coverage has added to the vocabulary of public health in recent years, "to promote and conduct research in the field of health" has always been central to WHO's goal of achieving "the highest attainable standard of health". **Chapter 5** briefly explains how WHO plays a role in both doing and supporting research through the Organization's Strategy on Research for Health. This report is closely aligned with the aims of the WHO strategy, which encourages the highest-quality research in order to deliver the greatest health benefits to the maximum number of people.

The role of research for
universal health coverage

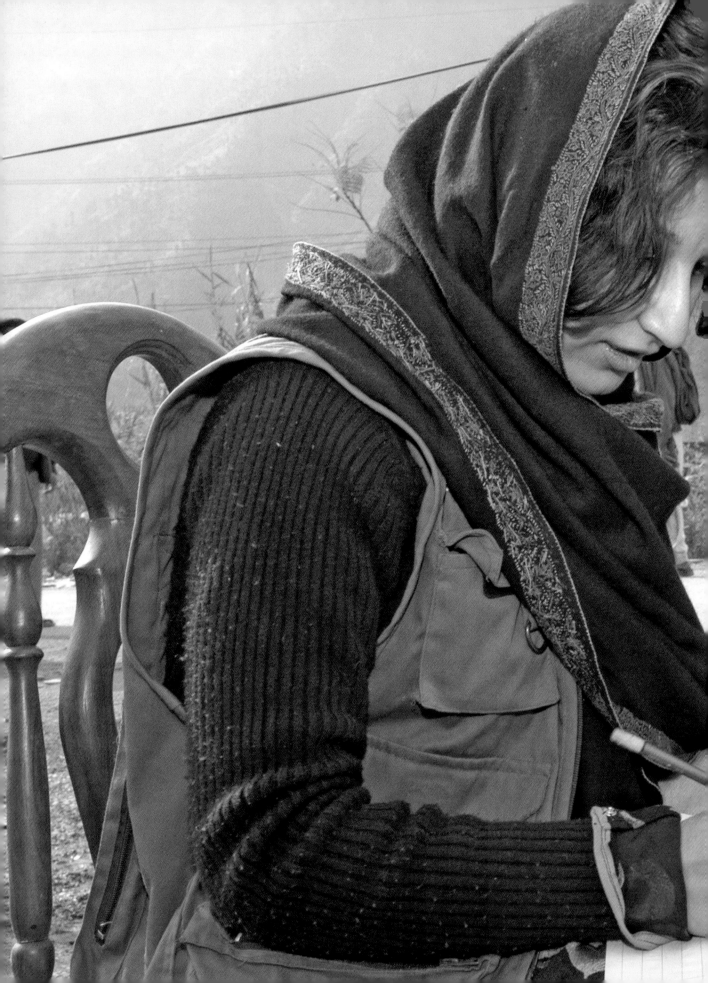

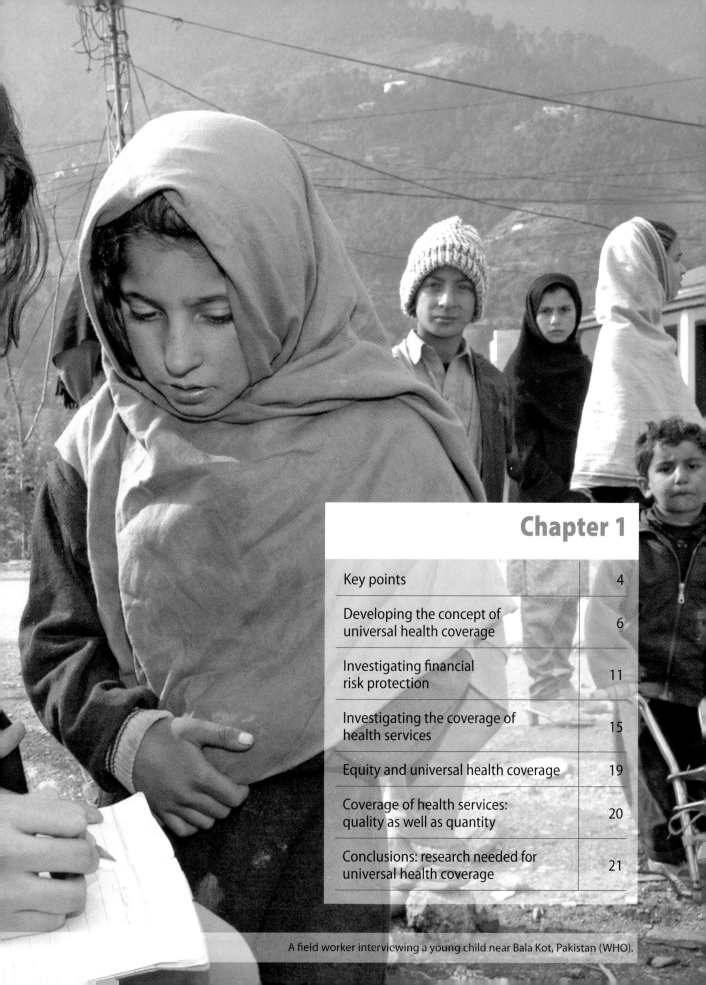

Chapter 1

A field worker interviewing a young child near Bala Kot, Pakistan (WHO).

Key points

- The goal of universal health coverage is to ensure that all people obtain the health services they need – prevention, promotion, treatment, rehabilitation and palliation – without risk of financial ruin or impoverishment, now and in the future.

- Since 2005, when all WHO Member States made the commitment to universal health coverage, many advances have been made in the provision of health services and in financial risk protection. This is illustrated by progress towards the health-related Millennium Development Goals (MDGs), and in the widespread fall in cash payments made for using health services.

- Despite this progress, the coverage of health services and financial risk protection currently fall far short of universal coverage. Thus nearly half of all HIV-infected people eligible for antiretroviral therapy were still not receiving it in 2011; and an estimated 150 million people suffer financial catastrophe each year because they have to pay out-of-pocket for health services.

- The conditions causing ill-health, and the financial capacity to protect people from ill-health, vary among countries. Consequently, given limited resources, each nation must determine its own priorities for improving health, the services that are needed, and the appropriate mechanisms for financial risk protection.

- These observations lead to research questions of two kinds. First, and most important, are questions about improving health and well-being – questions that help us to define the interventions and services that are needed, including financial risk protection, discover how to expand the coverage of these services, including the reduction of inequities in coverage, and investigate the effects of improved coverage on health. The second set of questions is about measurement – of the indicators and data needed to monitor service coverage, financial risk protection, and health impact. One task for research is to help define a set of common indicators for comparing progress towards universal coverage across all countries.

- Neither of these areas of questioning has permanent answers. Through the cycle of research – questions yield answers which provoke yet more questions – there will always be new opportunities to improve health. Today's targets for universal health coverage will inevitably be superseded in tomorrow's world of greater expectations.

1

The role of research for universal health coverage

The goal of universal health coverage is to ensure that everyone can use the health services they need without risk of financial ruin or impoverishment (*1*). As a descendant of the "Health for All" movement (Box 1.1), universal health coverage takes a broad view of the services that are needed for good health and well-being. These services range from clinical care for individual patients to the public services that protect the health of whole populations. They include services that come from both within and beyond the health sector. Financial risk protection is one element in the package of measures that provides overall social protection (*7*). And protection against severe financial difficulties in the event of illness gives the peace of mind that is an integral part of well-being.

To support the goal of universal health coverage is also to express concern for equity and for honouring everyone's right to health (*8*). These are personal and moral choices regarding the kind of society that people wish to live in, taking universal coverage beyond the technicalities of health financing, public health and clinical care.

With a greater understanding of the scope of universal health coverage, many national governments now view progress towards that goal as a guiding principle for the development of health systems, and for human development generally. It is clear that healthier environments mean healthier people (*9*). Preventive and curative services protect health and protect incomes (*10, 11*). Healthy children are better able to learn, and healthy adults are better able to contribute socially and economically.

The path to universal health coverage has been dubbed "the third global health transition", after the demographic and epidemiological transitions (*12*). Universal coverage is now an ambition for all nations at all stages of development. The timetable and priorities for action clearly differ between countries, but the higher aim of ensuring that all people can use the health services they need without risk of financial hardship is the same everywhere.

Box 1.1. From "Health for All" to universal health coverage

Universal health coverage is an aspiration that underpins "the enjoyment of the highest attainable standard of health" which, as stated in WHO's constitution, is "one of the fundamental rights of every human being without distinction of race, religion, political belief, economic or social condition" (2). To reach the highest attainable standard of health is an objective that has guided health policy nationally and internationally for 65 years, finding voice in WHO's "Health for All" programme which began in the 1970s and was enshrined in the Alma Ata Declaration of 1978.

The Alma Ata Declaration is best known for promoting primary health care as a means to address the main health problems in communities, fostering equitable access to promotive, preventive, curative, palliative and rehabilitative health services.

The idea that everyone should have access to the health services they need underpinned a resolution of the 2005 World Health Assembly, which urged Member States "to plan the transition to universal coverage of their citizens so as to contribute to meeting the needs of the population for health care and improving its quality, to reducing poverty, and to attaining internationally agreed development goals" (3).

The central role of primary care within health systems was reiterated in *The world health report 2008* which was devoted to that topic (4). *The world health report 2010* on health systems financing built on this heritage by proposing that health financing systems – which countries of all income levels constantly seek to modify and adapt – should be developed with the specific goal of universal health coverage in mind.

The twin goals of ensuring access to health services, plus financial risk protection, were reaffirmed in 2012 by a resolution of the United Nations General Assembly which promotes universal health coverage, including social protection and sustainable financing (5). The 2012 resolution goes even further; it highlights the importance of universal health coverage in reaching the MDGs, in alleviating poverty and in achieving sustainable development (6). It recognizes, as did the "Health for All" movement and the Alma Ata Declaration, that health depends not only on having access to medical services and a means of paying for these services, but also on understanding the links between social factors, the environment, natural disasters and health.

This brief history sets the scene for this report. *The world health report 2013: research for universal health coverage* addresses questions about prevention and treatment, about how services can be paid for by individuals and governments, about their impact on the health of populations and the health of individuals, and about how to improve health through interventions both within and beyond the health sector. Although the focus of universal health coverage is on interventions whose primary objective is to improve health, interventions in other sectors – agriculture, education, finance, industry, housing and others – may bring substantial health benefits.

Developing the concept of universal health coverage

The world health report 2010 represented the concept of universal health coverage in three dimensions: the health services that are needed, the number of people that need them, and the costs to whoever must pay – users and third-party funders (Fig. 1.1) (1, 13).

The health services include approaches to prevention, promotion, treatment, rehabilitation and palliative care, and these services must be sufficient to meet health needs, both in quantity and in quality. Services must also be prepared for the unexpected – environmental disasters, chemical or nuclear accidents, pandemics, and so on.

The need for financial risk protection is determined by the proportion of costs that individuals must themselves cover by making direct and immediate cash payments.[a] Under universal coverage, there would be no out-of-pocket payments that exceed a given threshold

---

[a] Indirect costs, due for example to lost earnings, are not considered to be part of financial risk protection, but are part of the larger goal of social protection.

Fig. 1.1.   Measuring progress towards universal health coverage in three dimensions

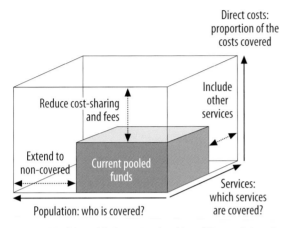

Source: World Health Organization (1) and Busse, Schreyögg & Gericke (13).

of affordability – usually set at zero for the poorest and most disadvantaged people. The total volume of the large box in Fig. 1.1 is the cost of all services for everyone at a particular point in time (1). The volume of the smaller blue box shows the health services and costs that are covered from pre-paid, pooled funds. The goal of universal coverage is for everyone to obtain the services they need at a cost that is affordable to themselves and to the nation as a whole.

All governments should therefore decide what health services are needed, and how to make sure they are universally available, affordable, efficient, and of good quality (14, 15). The services that are needed differ from one setting to another because the causes of ill-health also vary. The balance of services inevitably changes over time, as new technologies and procedures emerge as a result of research and innovation, following the changes in the causes of ill-health. In deciding which services to provide, institutions such as the National Institute for Health and Clinical Excellence (NICE) in England and Wales and the Health Intervention and Technology Assessment Programme (HITAP)

in Thailand (Box 1.2) have a vital role in evaluating whether interventions are effective and affordable.

In every country, there are people who are unable to pay directly, out-of-pocket, for the services they need, or who may be seriously disadvantaged by doing so. When people on low incomes with no financial risk protection fall ill they face a dilemma: if a local health service exists, they can decide to use the service and suffer further impoverishment in paying for it, or they can decide not to use the service, remain ill and risk being unable to work (20). The general solution for achieving wide coverage of financial risk protection is through various forms of prepayment for services. Prepayments allow funds to be pooled so that they can be redistributed to reduce financial barriers for those who need to use services they could not otherwise afford. This spreads the financial risks of ill-health across whole populations. Prepayment can be derived from taxation, other government charges or health insurance, and usually comes from a mixture of sources (1).

Financial risk protection of this kind is an instrument of social protection applied to health (7). It works alongside other mechanisms of social protection – unemployment and sickness benefits, pensions, child support, housing assistance, job-creation schemes, agricultural insurance and so on – many of which have indirect consequences for health.

Governments, especially in low-income countries, cannot usually raise sufficient funds by prepayment to eliminate excess out-of-pocket expenditures for all the health services that people need (1). It is therefore a challenge to decide how best to support health within budgetary limits. Fig. 1.1 offers three options for spending: maximize the proportion of the population covered by existing services, diversify health services by offering more types of intervention, or use the money for financial compensation, thereby reducing cash payments for health care.

Box 1.2. How Thailand assesses the costs and benefits of health interventions and technologies

In 2001 the Government of Thailand introduced universal health coverage financed from general taxation. Economic recession underlined the need for rigorous evaluation of health technologies that would be eligible for funding in order to prevent costs from escalating. At the time, no organization had the capacity to carry out the volume of health technology assessments (HTAs) demanded by the government. Therefore the Health Intervention and Technology Assessment Programme (HITAP, www.hitap.net) was set up to assess the costs, effectiveness and cost–effectiveness of health technologies – not only medications and medical procedures but also social interventions, public health measures and changes to the health system itself (*16, 17*).

Unlike the National Institute for Health and Clinical Excellence (NICE) in England and Wales, which evaluates existing interventions only, HITAP does primary research, including observational studies and randomized controlled trials, as well as systematic reviews and meta-analyses based on secondary literature analysis. Its output takes the form of formal presentations, discussion with technical and policy forums and academic publications.

One example of HITAP's work is in devising a screening strategy for cervical cancer which is caused by infection with the human papillomavirus (HPV) and is a major cause of morbidity and mortality among Thai women. Despite the introduction of Papanicolaou (Pap) screening at every hospital over 40 years ago, only 5% of women were screened. Visual inspection of the cervix with the naked eye after application with acetic acid (VIA) was introduced as an alternative in 2001 because it did not require cytologists. When HITAP's study began, both VIA and Pap smears were being offered to women in parallel and there was pressure from vaccine companies, international health agencies and nongovernmental organizations (NGOs) to introduce the new HPV vaccine (*18*).

The options considered by HITAP were conventional Pap screening, VIA, vaccination or a combination of Pap screening and VIA. Costs were calculated on the basis of estimated levels of participation and included costs to the health-care provider, costs for women attending screening and costs for those who were treated for cervical cancer. Potential benefits were analysed by using a model that estimated the number of women who would go on to develop cervical cancer in each scenario, and the impact on quality-adjusted life years (QALYs) was calculated by using data from a cohort of Thai patients.

The study concluded that the most cost-effective strategy was to offer VIA to women every five years between the ages of 30 and 45, followed by a Pap smear every five years for women aged between 50 and 60 years. The strategy would offer an additional 0.01 QALYs and a total cost saving of 800 Baht, when compared to doing nothing. Universal introduction of vaccination for 15-year-old girls without screening would result in a gain of 0.06 QALYs at a cost of 8000 Baht, and either VIA and Pap screening alone would have costs and benefits somewhere between the two amounts (*19*).

The approach recommended by HITAP was piloted in several provinces starting in 2009, and this has now been implemented nationally. The actual impact is currently being assessed.

HITAP attributes its success to several factors:

- the strong research environment in Thailand which, for instance, provides staff for HITAP and supports peer review of their recommendations;
- collegiate relationships with similar institutions in other countries, such as NICE in England and Wales;
- working with peers (HITAP meets with other Asian HTA institutions, and has formed an association with Japan, Malaysia and the Republic of Korea);
- transparency in research methods, so that difficult or unpopular decisions can be understood;
- a code of conduct (HITAP adheres to a strict code of behaviour which, for instance, precludes acceptance of gifts or money from pharmaceutical companies);
- political support from government, fostered by opening doors to, and discussing methods with, decision-makers;
- popular support, generated by lectures at universities and dissemination of recommendations to the general public;
- external review (HITAP commissioned an external review of its methods and work in 2009).

Fig. 1.2.   A representation of the results chain for universal health coverage, focusing on the outcomes

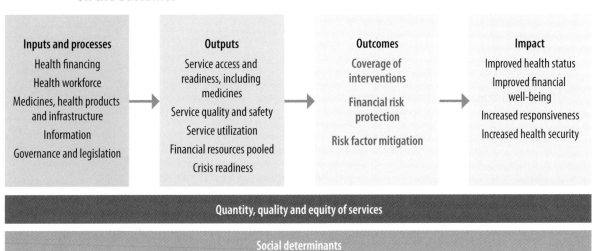

Inputs and processes	Outputs	Outcomes	Impact
Health financing	Service access and readiness, including medicines	Coverage of interventions	Improved health status
Health workforce	Service quality and safety	Financial risk protection	Improved financial well-being
Medicines, health products and infrastructure	Service utilization	Risk factor mitigation	Increased responsiveness
Information	Financial resources pooled		Increased health security
Governance and legislation	Crisis readiness		

Quantity, quality and equity of services

Social determinants

Note: Each of these outcomes depends on inputs, processes and outputs (to the left), and eventually makes an impact on health (to the right). Access to financial risk protection can also be considered an output. All measurements must reflect not only the quantity of services, but also quality and equity of access (first cross panel). Equity of coverage is influenced by "social determinants" (second cross panel), so it is vital to measure the spectrum from inputs to impact by income, occupation, disability, etc.

Financial investments are made in medicines and other commodities, as well as in infrastructure, in order to generate the services that have an impact on health. Fig. 1.2 is one way to portray this chain of events. Consider, for example, the links between tobacco smoking and health. The proportion of people who smoke in a population (outcome), which represents a risk factor for lung, heart and other diseases (impact), is affected by various services and policies that prevent ill-health and promote good health (outputs). Among these services and policies are face-to-face counselling, anti-smoking campaigns, bans on smoking in public places, and taxes on tobacco products. The population coverage achieved by these interventions, which are often used in combination, influences the number of smokers in the population (21).

In fact, the problem of tobacco smoking in relation to health goes beyond the results chain in Fig. 1.2. Smoking, like many other risk factors, tends to be more frequent among those who have had less formal education and who have

lower incomes. When seeking health care for smoking-related illnesses, people educated to a higher level are typically more aware of the services available and more disposed to use them. These "social determinants", which influence prevention and treatment of illness, are a reason for taking a broad view of research for health; they highlight the value of combining investigations both within and outside the health sector with the aim of achieving policies for "heath in all sectors" (Box 1.3 and Chapter 2).

Even with an understanding of the determinants and consequences of service coverage, the balancing of investments in health services is more than a technical matter. The allocation of public money to health also has ethical, moral and political implications. Public debate, based on evidence from research, is the mechanism for obtaining consensus on, for instance, who should be entitled to health care paid from the public purse, under what conditions, and for what range of services. Decisions on these issues, which involve a combination of ethical imperatives and political

Box 1.3. What do universal health coverage and social protection mean for people affected by tuberculosis?

Tuberculosis (TB) is a disease of poverty that drives people deeper into poverty (*22*). In recognition of this fact, TB diagnosis and treatment are free of charge for patients in most countries. The cost of TB treatment, provided as a public service, is covered by domestic health-care budgets, often supplemented by international grants or loans (*23*). This helps to reduce the financial barriers to accessing and adhering to treatment. However, free public health services are often not entirely free, and patients always face other expenses. Payments are made for medical tests, medicines, consultation fees and transport, and there are indirect costs of illness due to lost earnings.

For patients, therefore, the total cost of an episode of TB is often large in relation to their income (*24*). The average total cost incurred by TB patients in low- and middle-income countries has been estimated at between 20% and 40% of annual family income, and the relative cost is higher in the lower socioeconomic groups (*25–32*). The poorest patients become indebted: 40–70% of them according to three studies carried out in Africa and Asia (*26, 28, 29*). A large part of the cost of TB treatment is incurred during the diagnostic phase before treatment starts in a subsidized TB programme. Costs are especially high for diagnosis and treatment by private doctors, with whom many of the very poorest seek care first (*28, 29, 33, 34*). Financial costs are commonly compounded by adverse social consequences – such as rejection by family and friends, divorce, expulsion from school and loss of employment – which affect women in particular (*35–37*).

The research behind these findings has been essential for documenting the obstacles to the use of health services and the financial vulnerability of families affected by TB. It has helped to pinpoint where improved services, health insurance coverage and social protection can safeguard against the consequences of potentially fatal and financially catastrophic illness (*38*).

To estimate patients' costs and identify barriers to access, WHO and partners have developed a toolkit which has recently been field-tested in surveys in several countries. The results have begun to inform national policy on social protection for people with TB (*39, 40*). Beyond free diagnosis and treatment, a full package of measures for social protection requires the following:

- **Universal health care**, free of cost, or heavily subsidized. People do not enter the health-care system as TB patients eligible for free treatment; they typically enter as patients with a respiratory illness. The journey to correct diagnosis and the start of treatment often takes weeks or months. Out-of-pocket expenses need to be minimized across the health system (*23*).
- **Specific social or financial risk protection schemes**, compensating for the adverse financial or social effects of TB. For example, these may include travel vouchers, food packages, or cash transfers, as well as psychosocial support.
- **Legislation to protect workers**, ensuring that people with TB are not expelled from employment due to a disease that is normally rendered non-infectious after two weeks of correct treatment, and from which most patients fully recover.
- **Sickness insurance**, compensating income loss during illness.
- **Instruments to protect human rights**, minimizing stigma and discrimination, with special attention to gender, ethnicity and protection of the vulnerable groups that are at particularly high risk of TB.
- **Whole-of-government approaches to address social determinants of health**, and policies based on "heath in all sectors", taking a broad view of the drivers of TB epidemics (Chapter 2). Poverty-reduction strategies and financial safety nets help prevent TB on many levels. Most important for TB prevention are good living and working conditions and good nutrition. Basic education supports universal health coverage by enabling healthy lifestyle choices and informing health-care decisions.

continues ...

... continued

None of the above is specific to TB, but TB control programmes are among those affected by the presence or absence of health services and mechanisms for social protection. While disease-specific solutions can help partly and temporarily, universal health coverage, including social protection, is vital for sustained and effective TB control. Disease control programmes need to ensure that the patients they serve are eligible for, and actually receive, support from the general health services and not only from TB control programmes.

TB has close links with poverty and social vulnerability, and is one of the conditions that can function as a tracer for universal coverage. However, national TB control programmes need to add measures of financial risk protection to existing indicators of service coverage. Among the measurable indicators are the following:

Outcome
- **For coverage of health services:** TB diagnosis and treatment coverage (percentage of TB cases receiving proper care, and percentage successfully treated; see Fig. 1.5) and equity in coverage.
- **For financial risk protection:** Access to financial risk protection schemes (percentage of patients using existing schemes) and equity of access.

Impact
- **For financial risk protection:** Cost of TB illness to patients (percentage with catastrophic expenditure, data from surveys, using the tool to estimate patients' costs).
- **Combined for universal coverage, financial risk protection and addressing social determinants:** TB incidence, prevalence and death rates (from programme surveillance data, vital registration and population-based surveys).

possibilities, place constraints on the analysis of how to maximize health impact for the money spent.

In summary, the first challenge in moving towards universal health coverage is to define the services and supporting policies needed in any setting, including financial risk protection, the population that needs to use these services, and the cost. This requires an understanding of the causes of ill-health, the possible interventions, who currently has access to these services and who does not, and the extent of financial hardship incurred by paying out-of-pocket. Acting on behalf of their populations, governments must decide how to move closer to universal coverage with limited financial resources. The second challenge is to measure progress towards universal coverage, using valid indicators and

appropriate data. The two challenges go together, and research provides the evidence to address them both.

To highlight the role of research, the concepts of financial risk protection and health service coverage are expanded below, and the strengths and weaknesses of methods for tracking progress in each area are considered.

Investigating financial risk protection

It is significant that, at a time of widespread economic austerity, even high-income countries are struggling to maintain current health services and to make sure that everyone can afford to use them (*41, 42*). The question of how to provide and maintain financial risk protection is relevant everywhere.

Access to financial risk protection could be expressed as the number of people enrolled in some type of insurance scheme or covered by a tax-funded health service free at the point of use (43). In fact, financial risk protection is often more accurately judged by the adverse consequences for people who are not protected (Box 1.4). As an example, survey data for 92 countries (inhabited by 89% of the world's population) show that the annual incidence of catastrophic health expenditure is close to zero in countries with well-established social protection systems, but up to 11% in countries without such systems. In 37 of the 92 countries surveyed, the annual incidence of financial catastrophe exceeded 2%, and in 15 it was above 4%.

An indirect measure of (the lack of) financial risk protection is the ratio of out-of-pocket payments to total health expenditure (table in Box 1.4; Fig. 1.3). In 63 countries, most of them low-income countries where many people need financial risk protection, more than 40% of all health expenditure took the form of direct out-of-pocket payments. At the other end of the scale, in 62 countries less than 20% of health expenditure was out-of-pocket. Although the majority of the 62 are high-income countries, among them are Algeria, Bhutan, Cuba, Lesotho and Thailand. The governments of these countries have shown how, despite low average incomes, the poorest people can be protected from having to make disastrously large cash payments for health.

These surveys are also being used to track the progress being made in financial risk protection over time. Between 2005 and 2010 the proportion of health spending made through out-of-pocket payments fell, on average, in all but one WHO region (46). The exception was Africa, where the level remained stable. Twenty-three countries across all regions and income levels achieved a reduction of at least 25% in the proportion of

health spending made through out-of-pocket payments. Nevertheless, an estimated 150 million people suffered financial catastrophe in 2010, and 100 million people were pushed below the poverty line (poverty is defined in Box 1.4) because they had to pay out-of-pocket for health care (46).

These conclusions derive from two different ways of expressing financial risk protection; one uses a direct measure from primary survey data, the other uses an indirect measure derived from two different sets of surveys. Although the indicators differ, the results are similar. The data suggest, as a rule of thumb, that when out-of-pocket payments fall to or below 15–20% of total health expenditure, the incidence of financial catastrophe will be negligible (47, 48).

While these surveys give useful insights into financial risk protection, they raise further questions about the different ideas that underpin financial risk protection, and about the sources of data and methods of measurement. For instance, should the incidence of catastrophic expenditure and impoverishment be given equal weight in describing the extent of financial risk protection in a country? Is it better to improve financial risk protection on average, or to set a minimum level of protection for everyone? How does financial risk protection reflect the broader goal of social protection? What targets or milestones should be set for measures of financial risk protection until universal coverage is fully achieved? Which conditions of ill-health, perhaps with costly treatments, tend to fall outside national financial risk protection mechanisms and therefore result in financial impoverishment for households? Do any of these measures capture the value associated with peace-of-mind – the assurance that is conferred by accessible, affordable, and reliable health services? These are topics for further research, and in some cases public debate, on the mechanisms of financial risk protection, and on the methods of measurement.

Box 1.4.   Measuring financial risk protection

The measurement of financial risk protection should ideally capture the number of people enrolled in some kind of health insurance scheme and the number of people who are eligible to use – and able to afford – health services provided by government, private sector or civil society.

Direct and indirect indicators of financial risk protection

Direct indicators	Explanation
Incidence of catastrophic health expenditure due to out-of-pocket payments	The number of people or the proportion of the population at all income levels who spend a disproportionate share of their incomes on out-of-pocket payments each year. Financial catastrophe is defined as out-of-pocket expenditure exceeding 40% of household income net of subsistence needs.
Mean positive overshoot of catastrophic payments	Shows the average amount by which households affected by catastrophic expenditures pay more than the threshold used to define catastrophic health spending.
Incidence of impoverishment due to out-of-pocket payments	The number of people or proportion of the population pushed below the poverty line because of out-of-pocket payments. The poverty line is crossed when daily income falls below a locally-defined threshold, typically around US$1–2 per day. For people who are living near the poverty threshold, even small payments push them below the threshold.
Poverty gap due to out-of-pocket payments	The extent to which out-of-pocket health payments worsen a households' pre-existing level of poverty.
Indirect indicators	
Out-of-pocket payments as a share of total health expenditure	There is a high correlation between this indicator and the incidence of financial catastrophe.
Government health expenditure as a share of GDP	This recognizes that in all countries the poor need to be covered by financial risk protection from general government revenues; they are rarely all covered when this proportion is less than 5%.

GDP, gross domestic product; US$, United States dollars.

There are, however, some difficulties in determining who is actually financially protected and to what extent, as two examples will make clear. First, health insurance as such does not guarantee full financial risk protection. Many forms of insurance cover only a minimum set of services, so that those insured are still required to make out-of-pocket payments of different types, including informal cash payments (1). Second, government-financed services may be inadequate. For instance, they may not be available close to where they are needed, there may be too few health workers or no medicines, or the services may be perceived to be unsafe. In India, for example, everyone is eligible to use government health services, but direct out-of-pocket payments are still among the highest in the world (44).

By contrast, it is more straightforward, and often more precise, to measure the consequences for people who do not have financial risk protection. The table above describes four direct indicators and two indirect indicators of protection which can be measured by household expenditure surveys that include spending on health, as illustrated in the main text. The techniques used to measure these indicators are well established as a result of investment in relevant research, and the survey data are readily available (45). To assess inequalities in financial risk protection, these indicators can also be measured for different population groups, and can be stratified by income (or expenditure or wealth), place of residence, migrant status and so on.

Annual updates on the data and indicators that measure financial risk protection for all countries are reported in WHO's Global Health Expenditure Database (44).

Fig. 1.3. **Out-of-pocket expenditures on health as a percentage of total expenditure on health, 2013**

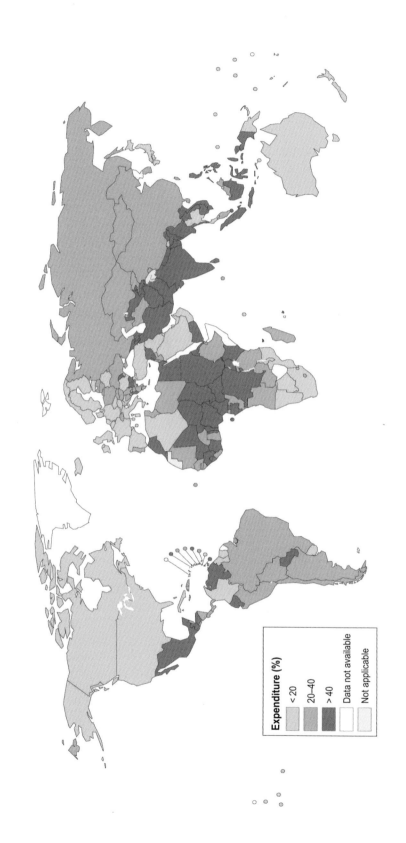

Expenditure (%)

< 20

20–40

> 40

Data not available

Not applicable

Note: Based on WHO data February 2013.

Investigating the coverage of health services

The evolution of thinking on universal health coverage has also led to a greater understanding of the functions that health systems should serve. These functions should be concerned with prevention as well as treatment. They should assure: (i) access to essential medicines and health products; (ii) motivated and skilled health workers who are accessible to the people they serve; (iii) integrated, high-quality, patient-centred services at all levels from primary to tertiary care; (iv) a combination of priority programmes for health promotion and disease control, including methods for prevention and treatment, which are integrated into health systems; (v) information systems that produce timely and accurate data for decision-making; and (vi) health financing systems that raise sufficient funds for health, provide financial risk protection, and ensure that funds are used equitably and efficiently.

In outlining the concept of universal coverage, Fig. 1.1 depicts health services along a single axis. In reality, there is a diversity of services delivered on several levels, depending on the nature of the health condition and the type of intervention. The elements of each row in Fig. 1.4 are the services that are deemed necessary. Preventive services (e.g. vaccines) and curative services (e.g. drug treatments) must address

Fig. 1.4.   A framework for measuring and monitoring the coverage of health services

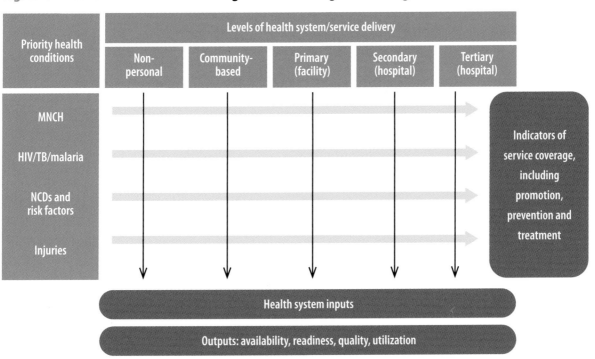

HIV, human immunodeficiency virus; MNCH, maternal, newborn and child health; NCDs, noncommunicable diseases; TB, tuberculosis.

Note: "Non-personal" health services are actions applied either to communities or populations – such as mass health education, policy development or taxation – or to the nonhuman components of the environment – such as environmental health measures. Community-based health services are defined as individual and community health actions delivered in the community (e.g. by community health workers) and not through health facilities. They are often considered to be part of the primary health care service.

the principal causes of ill-health now and in the future (e.g. the causes addressed by MDGs 4–6, and noncommunicable diseases in low-income countries). The columns in Fig. 1.4 represent the various levels on which services are delivered: in the community, to individuals at primary care centres or at secondary or tertiary hospitals, and to whole populations (nonpersonal) (49). As illustrated by its position in Fig. 1.4, a strong primary care system is central to an effective health system (4). "Nonpersonal" services are actions applied either to communities or to populations; broadly, they are educational, environmental, public health and policy measures in a range of sectors that influence health.

The MDGs have been a powerful force both for better health and for measuring progress towards better health with precisely-defined indicators, data collected in standard ways, and with internationally-agreed targets (46, 50). As an illustration, Fig. 1.5 shows some examples of progress towards MDG 6 (i.e. "to combat HIV/AIDS, malaria and other diseases"). For HIV/AIDS, "universal access" to antiretroviral therapy is currently defined as treatment of at least 80% of the eligible population. By 2010, 47% of eligible people were receiving treatment. Thus the target was missed globally, but national data show that it was reached in 10 countries, including some countries with a high prevalence of HIV, such as Botswana, Namibia and Rwanda.

MDG 7 is concerned with environmental sustainability. As a contribution to universal coverage, it includes the target to reduce by half, between 1990 and 2015, the proportion of people without access to safe drinking-water and basic sanitation. Notwithstanding some methodological limitations in measurement, more than two billion people gained access to improved drinking-water sources between 1990 and 2010, including piped supplies and protected wells. The MDG target was met by 2010, although access to improved water supplies was generally lower in rural areas than in urban ones (50, 55).

These investigations of progress towards the MDGs show, for selected interventions, how far we are from universal coverage. Ideally, we should measure the coverage of all the interventions that make up health services, but that is not usually possible even in high-income countries. In Mexico, for example, 472 interventions were covered by five separate health protection mechanisms in 2012, mainly under the health insurance programme known as *Seguro Popular* (Chapter 3, case-study 11) (43). It is feasible, however, to take a selection of interventions and indicators, and use them as "tracers" of the overall progress towards universal coverage. The interventions selected should be accessible to everyone who is eligible to receive them under universal health coverage in any setting.

Whether the tracers actually represent access to all health services needs to be evaluated, and this is a task for research. Nevertheless, to illustrate the idea, Box 1.5 shows how tracers of the coverage of maternal and child health services, combined with measures of financial risk protection, give an overview of service coverage in the Philippines and Ukraine. The two countries are similar with respect to the coverage of health services. The differences are in the incidence of catastrophic health expenditure and of poverty due to out-of-pocket payments.

An important function of this kind of analysis is to stimulate national policy dialogues about why the coverage of certain interventions is insufficient. For instance, in the comparison in Box 1.5, would the addition of other interventions tell a different story about progress towards universal coverage? Do the indicators of catastrophic expenditure and poverty represent aspects of financial risk protection that differ between the two countries? And there is always the question: "Are the underlying data accurate?"

The coverage of services depends on how those services are provided. The inputs can be investigated in addition to, or as a proxy for, direct measures of coverage (Fig. 1.2). For instance, WHO

Fig. 1.5.   Towards universal health coverage: examples of the growing coverage of interventions for the control of HIV/AIDS, tuberculosis, malaria and neglected tropical diseases

A. HIV/AIDS: coverage of antiretroviral therapy

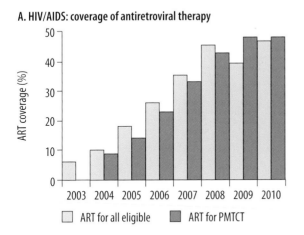

B. Tuberculosis: case detection and cure rates

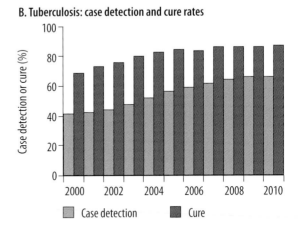

C. Malaria: vector control, diagnosis, treatment

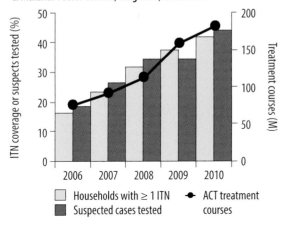

D. Neglected tropical diseases: preventive chemotherapy

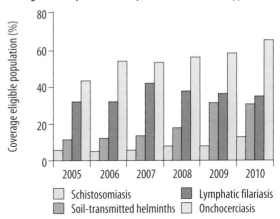

ACT, artemisinin-based combination therapies; AIDS, acquired immunodeficiency syndrome; ART, antiretroviral therapy; HIV, human immunodeficiency virus; ITN, insecticide-treated bed nets; PMTCT, prevention of mother-to-child transmission.

Note: Between 2003 and 2008, the denominator for ART coverage was all HIV-infected people with CD4 cell counts of ≤ 200 cells/µL, but in 2009 and 2010 the denominator was all people with ≤ 350 CD4 cells/µL. Hence the apparent fall in coverage between 2008 and 2009.

For PMTCT with ART, the numerator in 2010 excludes treatment with single-dose nevirapine.

For malaria, data on household coverage with ITN and on suspected cases tested are for the WHO African Region. Data on ACT are for the whole world.

The interpretation of universal coverage is 100% coverage for all interventions, except for interim targets of ≥ 80% coverage for ART, ≥ 90% for the percentage of tuberculosis patients cured, and variable coverage targets for neglected tropical diseases (*23, 51–53*). Reproduced, by permission of the publisher, from Dye et al. (*54*).

Box 1.5.   Measuring the coverage of health services

It is not usually possible to measure all aspects of service coverage even in high-income countries, but it is feasible to define a set of "tracer" conditions, with associated indicators and targets for interventions, to track progress towards universal coverage. The choice of tracer conditions and the associated indicators and data, and the work to demonstrate that these measures are representative and robust, are topics for further research (56).

Using tracers to track progress towards universal coverage in the Philippines and Ukraine

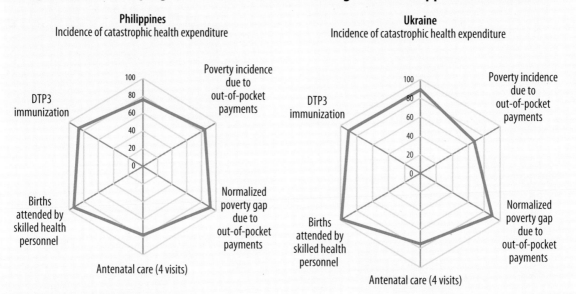

DTP3, diphtheria–tetanus–pertussis.

As an example, three tracers of the coverage of maternal and child health services, together with three measures of financial risk protection, give an overview of service coverage in the Philippines and Ukraine (see figure). The three service coverage indicators are: skilled birth attendants during delivery, three-dose diphtheria–tetanus–pertussis (DTP3) immunization and four antenatal visits (%). The three indicators of financial risk protection are: incidence of financial catastrophe due to direct out-of-pocket payments, incidence of impoverishment due to out-of-pocket payments, and the widening of the poverty gap due to out-of-pocket payments. For impoverishment, the worst possible outcome was estimated to be 5%, which is higher than measured impoverishment due to out-of-pocket payments in any country. In the figure, 100% service coverage and financial risk protection lie at the outer edge of the radar diagram, so a fully-filled polygon represents universal coverage. However, financial risk protection is measured as the consequences of its absence (Box 1.3), so the percentage scale is reversed for these three indicators.

With respect to the coverage of health services, the Philippines and Ukraine are similar. The differences are in the incidence of catastrophic health expenditure (higher in the Philippines) and the incidence of poverty due to out-of-pocket payments (higher in Ukraine). These observations, based on this particular set of indicators, raise questions about how to make further progress towards universal coverage (see main text).

These six tracers could be supplemented with others. For instance, standard indicators of progress exist for HIV/AIDS, tuberculosis, malaria, and some noncommunicable conditions (Fig. 1.5) (57). As more indicators are added, the polygon in the figure approaches a circle. Ideally, all indicators would be disaggregated by wealth quintile, place of residence, disability and gender, and by other important characteristics of population groups.

Fig. 1.6.   Availability of selected generic medicines in public and private health facilities during the period 2007–2011

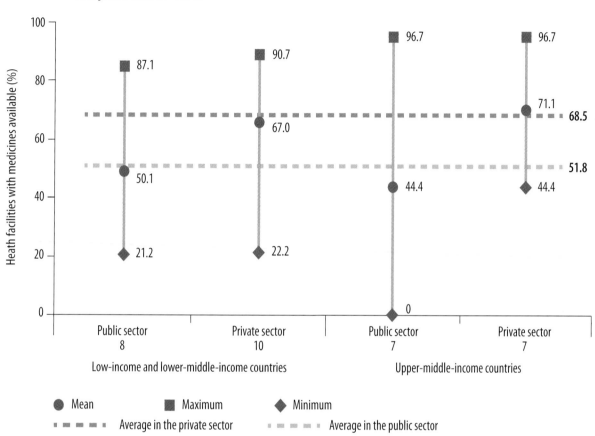

Reproduced, by permission of the publisher, from United Nations (*58*).

compiles data from surveys of the availability and price of essential medicines (Fig. 1.6) (*58*). Surveys carried out between 2007 and 2011 found that 14 generic essential medicines were available on average in 52% of public health facilities and in 69% of private health facilities. The averages differed little between lower-middle-income countries and upper-middle-income countries, and there were large variations among countries within each category. Among upper-middle-income countries, the availability of the 14 generic medicines varied from zero in the State of Rio Grande do Sul, Brazil, to 97% in the Islamic Republic of Iran.

One advantage of monitoring essential medicines as one way of tracking service coverage is that comparable data are increasingly available, and the quality of these data, collected through regular health facility assessments, is also improving. More than 130 countries had an essential medicines list by 2007, and 81% of the low-income countries had updated their lists in the previous five years.

Equity and universal health coverage

Systems for monitoring the coverage of services should record not only the total number of people who have or do not have access, but also some sociodemographic details about them. When coverage is truly universal everyone has access, but partial coverage may benefit certain groups over others. To monitor equity in the supply of, and demand for, health services, indicators should be disaggregated by income or wealth, sex, age, disability, place of residence (e.g. rural/urban, province or district), migrant status and ethnic origin (e.g. indigenous groups). For instance, gains in access to safe drinking-water have been uneven: 19% of people living in rural areas did not have improved water sources by 2010, in contrast with only 4% in urban areas (*50*). This analysis shows where to target further efforts to improve coverage.

Another example of the uneven distribution of services – for maternal, newborn and child health – is portrayed in Fig. 1.7. The summary measure of service coverage includes family planning, maternal and newborn care, childhood vaccination, and treatment of childhood illness. The mean coverage in 46 low- and middle-income countries varied by wealth quintile as expected, but there was also great variation within each quintile. To achieve universal health coverage, it is necessary to eliminate the gap between the poorest and richest both within and between quintiles, and to raise the levels in all quintiles. As a general rule, the countries that make the greatest progress in maternal and child health are those that successfully narrow the gap between the poorest and richest quintiles (*59, 60*). This is a form of "progressive universalism" in which the poorest individuals gain at least as much as the richest on the way to universal coverage (*61*).

Coverage of health services: quality as well as quantity

It is not just the quantity of health services provided that is important, but also the quality of them. Following a long tradition of research on the quality of care, the Organisation for Economic Co-operation and Development (OECD) has developed measures of quality for selected interventions: for cancer and mental

Fig. 1.7. **A summary measure of service coverage for maternal and child health, in which inequity is reflected in the differences between wealth quintiles**

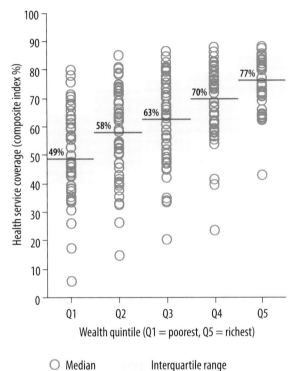

Source: Demographic and Health Surveys or Multiple Indicator Cluster Surveys in 46 low- and middle-income countries.

health, for aspects of prevention and health promotion, and for patient safety and patient experiences (*15, 62–64*).

Fig. 1.8 illustrates one aspect of the quality of care, namely the risk of death in hospital following ischaemic stroke. The risk is measured as the proportion of people who die within 30 days of admission (Fig. 1.8) (*65*). As with many measures of quantity, national statistics on the quality of care are often not precisely comparable. In this instance, case-fatality rates should ideally be based on individual patients, but some national databases do not track patients in and out of hospitals, between hospitals or even within the same hospital, because they do not

Fig. 1.8.   Case-fatality rates following ischaemic stroke during the 30 days after admission to hospitals in OECD countries for which there are data

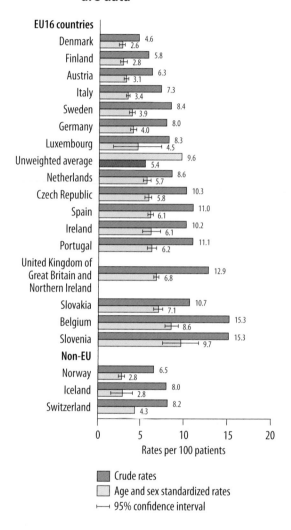

EU, European Union.
Note: Rates are standardized by age and sex to the entire 2005 OECD population aged ≥ 45 years.
Reproduced, by permission of the publisher, from the Organisation for Economic Co-operation and Development (65).

use unique patient identifiers. The data in Fig. 1.8 are therefore based on single hospital admissions and are restricted to mortality within the same hospital. There are big differences in case-fatality rates between countries, but some of the variation might be explained by local practices of discharging patients from hospitals, and transferring patients to other hospitals. To select and agree on internationally comparable indicators of quality is another task for research.

Conclusions: research needed for universal health coverage

When all WHO Member States made a commitment to achieving universal health coverage in 2005 they took a major step forward for public health. Taking that step launched an agenda for research. We do not yet know how to ensure that everyone has access to all the health services they need in all settings, and there are many gaps in understanding the links between service coverage and health (66, 67). Research is the means of filling these gaps.

With a focus on research, the goal of this report is not to measure definitively the gap between the present coverage of health services and universal coverage, but rather to identify the questions that arise as we try to achieve universal coverage and to discuss how these questions can be answered in order to accelerate progress.

In this chapter research questions of two kinds have been identified. The first and most important set of questions is about choosing the health services needed, improving the coverage of those services and of financial risk protection, and assessing the way in which greater coverage of both leads to better health and well-being. The second set of questions concerns measurement of the indicators and data that are needed to monitor coverage, financial risk protection, and the benefits for health.

The health services that are necessary and the people who need them should be defined with respect to the causes of ill-health, the technologies and instruments for intervention, and the cost. The services required vary from one setting to another, as does the capacity to pay for them. The function of research is to investigate whether schemes devised to achieve universal health coverage really succeed in their aims. At present the evidence on this issue is mixed. A comparative study of 22 low- and middle-income countries found that interventions to support universal health coverage usually improve access to health care. The study also found, less convincingly, that such interventions can have a positive effect on financial risk protection and, in some instances, a positive impact on health (68). Another conclusion of the review was that the effects of interventions varied according to the context, design and process of implementation. Such variation is illustrated further in Chapter 3 of this report.

The second set of questions about measurement is instrumental to answering the first set. Just as the necessary health services vary between settings, so too must the combination of indicators for measuring the coverage of services. Because it is not possible to measure the coverage of all services, a set of tracer interventions can be selected, with their associated indicators, to represent the overall quantity and quality of health services. The tracer conditions could be selected to exemplify major types of diseases or health problems such as acute infections, chronic infections and noncommunicable diseases. Universal coverage is achieved when each intervention is accessible to all who need it, and when it has the intended effects. Although every country has its own priorities for improving health, it would be possible, in principle, to choose a set of common indicators for comparing progress towards universal coverage across all countries. To define such a set of indicators is another task for research.

There are already numerous indicators of health-service coverage that have been standardized and validated, and they are widely used. The techniques for measurement have been greatly enhanced by tracking progress towards the MDGs, especially in low- and middle-income countries (50). However, beyond the MDGs there is less experience in monitoring prevention and control in other areas of health, such as noncommunicable diseases, ageing, and rehabilitation and palliative care (57). Similarly, while there are some standard indicators of the quality of health services, of equity of access, and of financial risk protection, there is much scope for refining the methods of data collection and measurement.

Universal health coverage is seen as a means of both improving health and promoting human development. This puts research for universal coverage in the wider context of research for development. Research will play a role not only in meeting the MDGs but also in supporting the post-2015 development agenda. For example, more research is needed to improve the resilience of health systems to environmental threats such as those posed by climate change. An additional and complementary challenge to that of increasing universal health coverage is to develop research that can enhance understanding of how intersectoral policies can improve health and advance development.

Because many more questions can be asked than answered, it is vital to set priorities for investigation. Research needs researchers with skill and integrity, who are funded to work in well-equipped institutions. Further, to make sure that research delivers results that lead to improvements in health, mechanisms are needed to translate evidence into action.

These elements of a successful research system are described more fully in Chapter 4. Before that, Chapter 2 highlights some of the recent developments in research for health worldwide; these provide the basis on which to build better research systems. Chapter 3 shows, by example, how research can address a wide range of questions about universal health coverage and how it can provide answers to guide health policy and practice. ■

References

1. *The world health report 2010. Health systems financing: the path to universal coverage.* Geneva, World Health Organization, 2010.
2. *Constitution of the World Health Organization.* Geneva, World Health Organization, 2006.
3. Resolution WHA58.33. Sustainable health financing, universal coverage and social health insurance. In: *Fifty-eighth World Health Assembly, Geneva, 16–25 May 2005. Volume 1. Resolutions and decisions.* Geneva, World Health Organization, 2005 (Document WHA58/2005/REC/1).
4. *The world health report 2008 – primary health care, now more than ever.* Geneva, World Health Organization, 2008.
5. United Nations General Assembly Resolution A/RES/67/81. *Global health and foreign policy.* Sixty-seventh session. Agenda item 123, 2012.
6. Evans DB, Marten R, Etienne C. Universal health coverage is a development issue. *Lancet*, 2012,380:864-865. doi: http://dx.doi.org/10.1016/S0140-6736(12)61483-4 PMID:22959373
7. *World social security report 2010/11. Providing coverage in times of crisis and beyond.* Geneva, International Labour Office, 2010.
8. Chan M. *Address at the Conference of Ministers of Finance and Health. Achieving value for money and accountability for health outcomes, Tunis, 4 July 2012.* (http://www.who.int/dg/speeches/2012/tunis_20120704, accessed 7 March 2013).
9. Haines A et al. From the Earth Summit to Rio+20: integration of health and sustainable development. *Lancet*, 2012,379:2189-2197. doi: http://dx.doi.org/10.1016/S0140-6736(12)60779-X PMID:22682465
10. Foster A. Poverty and illness in low-income rural areas. *The American Economic Review*, 1994,84:216-220.
11. Bloom DE, Canning D. The health and wealth of nations. *Science*, 2000,287:1207-1209. doi: http://dx.doi.org/10.1126/science.287.5456.1207 PMID:10712155
12. Rodin J, de Ferranti D. Universal health coverage: the third global health transition? *Lancet*, 2012,380:861-862. doi: http://dx.doi.org/10.1016/S0140-6736(12)61340-3 PMID:22959371
13. Busse R, Schreyögg J, Gericke C. *Analysing changes in health financing arrangements in high-income countries. A comprehensive framework approach.* Washington, DC, The World Bank, 2007.
14. Chisholm D, Evans DB. *Improving health system efficiency as a means of moving towards universal coverage.* Geneva, World Health Organization, 2010.
15. *Improving value in health care: measuring quality.* Paris, Organisation for Economic Co-operation and Development, 2010.
16. Tantivess S, Teerawattananon Y, Mills A. Strengthening cost-effectiveness analysis in Thailand through the establishment of the health intervention and technology assessment program. *PharmacoEconomics*, 2009,27:931-945. doi: http://dx.doi.org/10.2165/11314710-000000000-00000 PMID:19888793
17. Hanson K et al. Scaling up health policies and services in low- and middle-income settings. *BMC Health Services Research*, 2010,10:Suppl 1:I1. doi: http://dx.doi.org/10.1186/1472-6963-10-S1-I1 PMID:20594366
18. Yothasamut J et al. Scaling up cervical cancer screening in the midst of human papillomavirus vaccination advocacy in Thailand. *BMC Health Services Research*, 2010,10:Suppl 1:S5. doi: http://dx.doi.org/10.1186/1472-6963-10-S1-S5 PMID:20594371
19. Praditsitthikorn N et al. Economic evaluation of policy options for prevention and control of cervical cancer in Thailand. *PharmacoEconomics*, 2011,29:781-806. doi: http://dx.doi.org/10.2165/11586560-000000000-00000 PMID:21838332
20. McIntyre D, et al . What are the economic consequences for households of illness and of paying for health care in low- and middle-income country contexts? *Social Science & Medicine*, 2006,62:858-865. doi: http://dx.doi.org/10.1016/j.socscimed.2005.07.001 PMID:16099574
21. *WHO report on the global tobacco epidemic, 2011: warning about the dangers of tobacco.* Geneva, World Health Organization, 2011.
22. Lönnroth K et al. Drivers of tuberculosis epidemics: the role of risk factors and social determinants. *Social Science & Medicine*, 2009,68:2240-2246. doi: http://dx.doi.org/10.1016/j.socscimed.2009.03.041 PMID:19394122
23. *Global tuberculosis report 2012.* Geneva, World Health Organization, 2012. (http://www.who.int/tb/publications/global_report, accessed 24 March 2013).
24. Barter DM et al. Tuberculosis and poverty: the contribution of patient costs in sub-Saharan Africa – a systematic review. *BMC Public Health*, 2012,12:980. doi: http://dx.doi.org/10.1186/1471-2458-12-980 PMID:23150901
25. *Reaching the poor: challenges for TB programmes in the Western Pacific Region.* Manila, World Health Organization, 2004.
26. Hanson C, Weil D, Floyd K. Tuberculosis in the poverty alleviation agenda. In: Raviglione MC, ed. *Tuberculosis a comprehensive, international approach*, 3rd ed. New York, NY, CRC Press, 2006.
27. Kamolratanakul P et al. Economic impact of tuberculosis at the household level. *The International Journal of Tuberculosis and Lung Disease*, 1999,3:596-602. PMID:10423222

28. Rajeswari R et al. Socio-economic impact of tuberculosis on patients and family in India. *The International Journal of Tuberculosis and Lung Disease*, 1999,3:869-877. PMID:10524583

29. Wyss K, Kilima P, Lorenz N. Costs of tuberculosis for households and health care providers in Dar es Salaam, Tanzania. *Tropical Medicine & International Health*, 2001,6:60-68. doi: http://dx.doi.org/10.1046/j.1365-3156.2001.00677.x PMID:11251897

30. Lönnroth K et al. Social franchising of TB care through private GPs in Myanmar: an assessment of treatment results, access, equity and financial protection. *Health Policy and Planning*, 2007,22:156-166. doi: http://dx.doi.org/10.1093/heapol/czm007 PMID:17434870

31. Kemp JR et al. Can Malawi's poor afford free tuberculosis services? Patient and household costs associated with tuberculosis diagnosis in Lilongwe. *Bulletin of the World Health Organization*, 2007,85:580-585. doi: http://dx.doi.org/10.2471/BLT.06.033167 PMID:17768515

32. Pantoja A et al. Economic evaluation of public-private mix for tuberculosis care and control, India. Part I. Socio-economic profile and costs among tuberculosis patients. *The International Journal of Tuberculosis and Lung Disease*, 2009,13:698-704. PMID:19460244

33. Floyd K et al. Cost and cost-effectiveness of PPM-DOTS for tuberculosis control: evidence from India. *Bulletin of the World Health Organization*, 2006,84:437-445. doi: http://dx.doi.org/10.2471/BLT.05.024109 PMID:16799727

34. Uplekar M et al. Tuberculosis patients and practitioners in private clinics in India. *The International Journal of Tuberculosis and Lung Disease*, 1998,2:324-329. PMID:9559404

35. Porter JDH, Grange JM, eds. *Tuberculosis: an interdisciplinary perspective*. London, Imperial College Press, 1999.

36. Long NH. *Gender specific epidemiology of tuberculosis in Vietnam*. Stockholm, Karolinska Institutet, 2000.

37. Diwan V, Thorson A, Winkvist A. *Gender and tuberculosis*. Göteborg, Nordic School of Public Health, 1998.

38. Ananthakrishnan R et al. Expenditure pattern for TB treatment among patients registered in an urban government DOTS program in Chennai City, South India. *Tuberculosis Research and Treatment*, 2012,2012:747924. doi: http://dx.doi.org/10.1155/2012/747924 PMID:23213507

39. *Tool to estimate patients' costs*. Geneva, Stop TB Partnership, 2012. (http://www.stoptb.org/wg/dots_expansion/tbandpoverty/spotlight.asp, accessed 7 March 2013).

40. Mauch V et al. Free TB diagnosis and treatment are not enough - patient cost evidence from three continents. *The International Journal of Tuberculosis and Lung Disease*, 2013,17:381-387. doi: http://dx.doi.org/10.5588/ijtld.12.0368 PMID:23407227

41. Mladovsky P et al. *Health policy responses to the financial crisis in Europe*. Copenhagen, World Health Organization on behalf of the European Observatory on Health Systems and Policies, 2012.

42. Scherer P, Devaux M. *The challenge of financing health care in the current crisis. An analysis based on the OECD data*. Paris, Organisation for Economic Co-operation and Development, 2010 (OECD Health Working Papers, No. 49).

43. Knaul FM et al. The quest for universal health coverage: achieving social protection for all in Mexico. *Lancet*, 2012,380:1259-1279. doi: http://dx.doi.org/10.1016/S0140-6736(12)61068-X PMID:22901864

44. *Global health expenditure database*. Geneva, World Health Organization, 2012. (apps.who.int/nha/database/DataExplorerRegime.aspx, accessed 7 March 2013).

45. *ADePT: STATA software platform for automated economic analysis*. Washington, DC, The World Bank, 2012. (web.worldbank.org, accessed 24 March 2013).

46. *World health statistics 2012*. Geneva, World Health Organization, 2012.

47. Xu K et al. Protecting households from catastrophic health spending. *Health Affairs (Project Hope)*, 2007,26:972-983. doi: http://dx.doi.org/10.1377/hlthaff.26.4.972 PMID:17630440

48. Xu K et al. *Exploring the thresholds of health expenditure for protection against financial risk*. Geneva, World Health Organization, 2010 (World Health Report [2010] Background Paper, No 19).

49. *Measurement of trends and equity in coverage of health interventions in the context of universal health coverage. Rockefeller Foundation Center, Bellagio, September 17–21, 2012*. UHC Forward, 2012 (http://uhcforward.org/publications/measurement-trends-and-equity-coverage-health-interventions-context-universal-health-co, accessed 7 March 2013).

50. *The Millennium Development Goals report 2012*. New York, United Nations, 2012.

51. *Global report. UNAIDS report on the global AIDS epidemic*. Geneva, Joint United Nations Programme on HIV/AIDS, 2012.

52. *World malaria report 2012*. Geneva, World Health Organization, 2012.

53. *Sustaining the drive to overcome the global impact of neglected tropical diseases*. Geneva, World Health Organization, 2013.

54. Dye C et al. WHO and the future of disease control programmes. *Lancet*, 2013,381:413-418. doi: http://dx.doi.org/10.1016/S0140-6736(12)61812-1 PMID:23374479

55. United Nations Secretary General's Advisory Board on Water and Sanitation. *Monitoring and reporting progress of access to water & sanitation. An assessment by* UNSGAB. New York, United Nations, 2008.

56. Scheil-Adlung X, Florence B. Beyond legal coverage: assessing the performance of social health protection. *International Social Security Review*, 2011,64:21-38. doi: http://dx.doi.org/10.1111/j.1468-246X.2011.01400.x

57. Angell SY, Danel I, DeCock KM. Global indicators and targets for noncommunicable diseases. *Science*, 2012,337:1456-1457. doi: http://dx.doi.org/10.1126/science.1228293 PMID:22997310

58. *Millennium Development Goal 8. The global partnership for development: making rhetoric a reality.* New York, United Nations, 2012 (MDG Gap Task Force report 2012).

59. Victora CG et al. How changes in coverage affect equity in maternal and child health interventions in 35 Countdown to 2015 countries: an analysis of national surveys. *Lancet*, 2012,380:1149-1156. doi: http://dx.doi.org/10.1016/S0140-6736(12)61427-5 PMID:22999433

60. Ruhago GM, Ngalesoni FN, Norheim OF. Addressing inequity to achieve the maternal and child health millennium development goals: looking beyond averages. *BMC Public Health*, 2012,12:1119. doi: http://dx.doi.org/10.1186/1471-2458-12-1119 PMID:23270489

61. Gwatkin DR, Ergo A. Universal health coverage: friend or foe of health equity? *Lancet*, 2011,377:2160-2161. doi: http://dx.doi.org/10.1016/S0140-6736(10)62058-2 PMID:21084113

62. Donabedian A. The quality of care. How can it be assessed? *Journal of the American Medical Association*, 1988,260:1743-1748. doi: http://dx.doi.org/10.1001/jama.1988.03410120089033 PMID:3045356

63. Donabedian A. Evaluating the quality of medical care. *The Milbank Quarterly*, 2005,83:691-729. doi: http://dx.doi.org/10.1111/j.1468-0009.2005.00397.x PMID:16279964

64. Davies H. *Measuring and reporting the quality of health care: issues and evidence from the international research literature.* Edinburgh, NHS Quality Improvement Scotland, 2005.

65. *Health at a glance: Europe 2012.* Paris, Organisation for Economic Co-operation and Development, 2012. http://dx.doi.org/10.1787/9789264183896-en

66. Moreno-Serra R, Smith PC. Does progress towards universal health coverage improve population health? *Lancet*, 2012,380:917-923. doi: http://dx.doi.org/10.1016/S0140-6736(12)61039-3 PMID:22959388

67. Acharya A et al. *Impact of national health insurance for the poor and the informal sector in low- and middle-income countries: a systematic review.* London, EPPI-Centre, Social Science Research Unit, Institute of Education, University of London, 2012.

68. Giedion U, Alfonso EA, Díaz Y. *The impact of universal coverage schemes in the developing world: a review of the existing evidence.* Washington, DC, The World Bank, 2013.

The growth of research for
universal health coverage

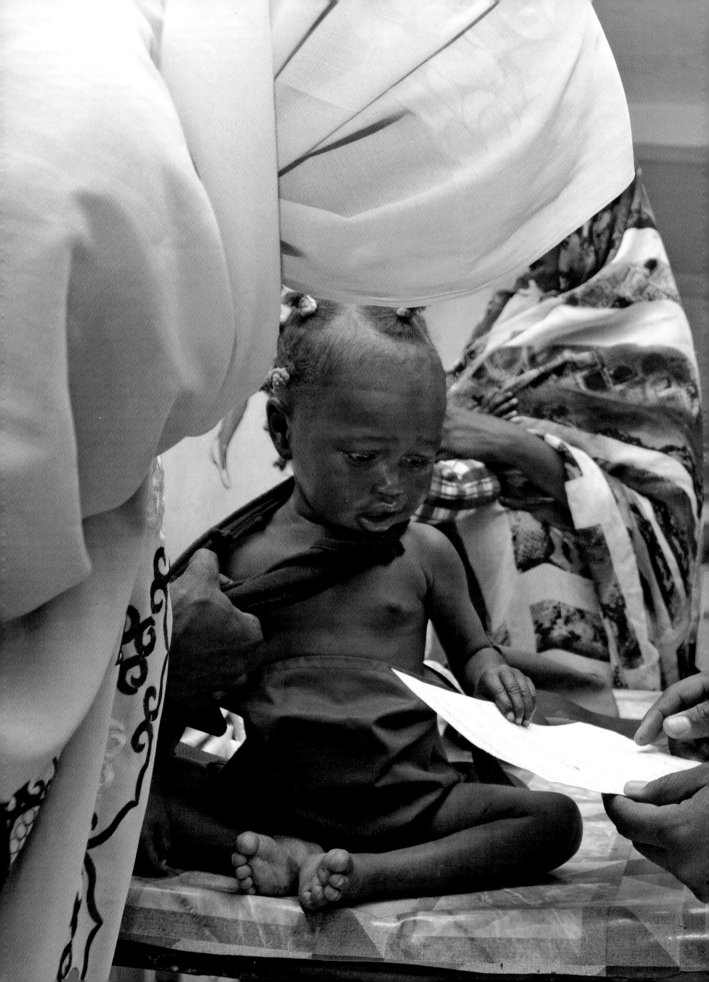

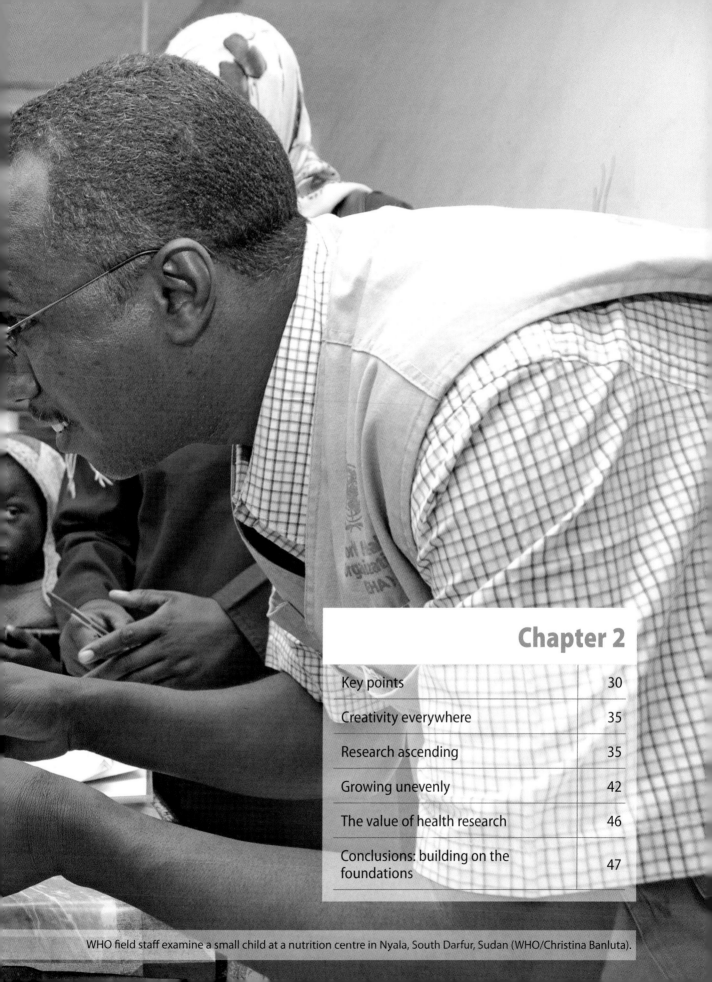

Chapter 2

WHO field staff examine a small child at a nutrition centre in Nyala, South Darfur, Sudan (WHO/Christina Banluta).

Key points

- Chapter 1 considered ways of measuring the gap between the present coverage and universal coverage of health services. The question of how to fill that gap is a target for research in every country. Research for universal health coverage, underpinned by research for health, is the body of methods and results used to find new ways of providing the health care needed by everyone.

- There are plenty of creative ideas about how to achieve comprehensive health care. They come from both within the health sector and beyond it and will flourish wherever they are permitted and encouraged to do so.

- Research to stimulate and harness new ideas is growing worldwide. The growth is uneven, but most countries now have the foundations on which to build effective research programmes.

- Not only is more research being done, it is also being done in more creative ways. One example is new thinking to break the mould of traditional research and development (R&D), where more products are being created through partnerships between universities, governments, international organizations and the private sector.

- The results of some research studies are widely applicable, but many questions about universal health coverage need local answers. All nations therefore need to be producers of research as well as consumers of it.

- In low- and middle-income countries, the principal challenges are to strengthen research systems, identify key research questions, and generate the capacity to turn research into practical applications.

- Research is in the ascendant, but few countries have objectively assessed the strengths and weaknesses of their national research programmes, and few have evaluated the health, social and economic benefits that research can bring. All nations will benefit from taking a systematic approach to the monitoring and evaluation of research investments, practices, outputs and applications.

2

The growth of research for universal health coverage

Chapter 1 defined universal health coverage and discussed practical ways to measure progress towards this goal. The discussion led to research questions of two kinds. The first kind is about improving health: What kinds of health systems and services are needed and for whom? How can the necessary health services be provided, and at what cost? How should health services adapt to the expected shifts in disease burden in the coming years?

The second kind of question is about measurement: What is the best way to measure the coverage of services and financial risk protection in any setting? How will we know when we have reached universal coverage?

In the context of this report, scientific research provides the set of tools used to stimulate and harness creative solutions to these questions – i.e. research gives us the formal techniques that turn promising ideas into practical methods for achieving universal health coverage.

This chapter gives an overview of the changing landscape of research. The first observation is that creativity, imagination and innovation – which are fundamental in any culture of enquiry – are universal. A premise of this report is that new ideas will flourish wherever they are encouraged and permitted to do so.

The second observation is that there has been a striking increase in research productivity in low- and middle-income countries over the past two decades, in the wake of the 1990 report of the Commission on Health Research for Development among others (1). A greater recognition of the value of research for health, society and the economy has added impetus to the upward trend. Although the growth is uneven, most countries now have the foundations on which to build effective research programmes.

The process of doing research presents questions on several levels: What health problem needs to be solved? On the spectrum from disease etiology to health policy, what kind of question is being asked about this problem?

The sequence of research questions is not linear but cyclical: questions lead to answers and then to yet more questions. For instance, which stages of investigation in the research cycle will be included – measuring the problem, understanding the options to address the problem, solving the problem by comparing the options, implementing the preferred solution, or evaluating the

Box 2.1.   Research definitions used in this report

Research is the development of knowledge with the aim of understanding health challenges and mounting an improved response to them (*2, 3*). Research is a vital source, but not the only source, of information that is used to develop health policy. Other considerations – cultural values, human rights, social justice and so on – are used to weigh the importance of different kinds of evidence in decision-making (*4, 5*).

Research excludes routine testing and routine analysis of technologies and processes, as would be done for the maintenance of health or disease control programmes, and as such is distinct from research to develop new analytical techniques. It also excludes the development of teaching materials that do not embody original research.

Basic research or **fundamental research** is experimental or theoretical work undertaken primarily to acquire new knowledge about the underlying foundations of phenomena and observable facts, without any particular application or use in view (*6*).

Applied research is original investigation undertaken to acquire new knowledge, directed primarily towards a specific practical aim or objective (*6*).

Operational research or **implementation research** seeks knowledge on interventions, strategies or tools so as to enhance the quality or coverage of health systems and services (*7, 8*). The design could be, for example, an observational study, a cross-sectional study, a case–control or cohort study, or a randomized controlled trial (Box 2.3).

Translational research, which moves knowledge gained from basic research to its application in the clinic and community, is often characterized as "bench-to-bedside" and "bedside-to-community". The translation is between any of several stages: moving basic discovery into a candidate health application; assessing the value of an application leading to the development of evidence-based guidelines; moving guidelines into health practice, through delivery, dissemination, and diffusion research; or evaluating the health outcomes of public health practice (*9*). This has also been called **experimental development research**, which is the terminology used in the study described in Fig. 2.3.

Health policy and systems research (HPSR) seeks to understand and improve how societies organize themselves in achieving their collective health goals, and how different actors interact in the policy and implementation processes to contribute to policy outcomes. HPSR is an interdisciplinary blend of economics, sociology, anthropology, political science, public health and epidemiology that together draw a comprehensive picture of how health systems respond and adapt to health policies, and how health policies can shape – and be shaped by – health systems and the broader determinants of health (*10*).

Research for health covers a broader range of investigations than **health research**, reflecting the fact that health also depends on actions taken outside the health sector – in agriculture, education, employment, fiscal policy, housing, social services, trade, transport and so on. This wider view of research will become increasingly important in the transition from the United Nations Millennium Development Goals to a post-2015 sustainable development agenda. As pointed out in Box 1.1, research for universal health coverage is also research for development.

Research for universal health coverage, which is a part of all research for health, is the body of questions, methods and results used to find new ways of providing the health care that is needed by everyone.

Innovation is a general term referring to the introduction of something new – an idea, a strategy, a method or a device. New ideas can be objectively evaluated by the research process.

outcome? Along the gradient from observational studies (typically weaker inferences) to randomized controlled trials (stronger inferences), what study designs will be used? In parallel to the main narrative of this chapter, three accompanying boxes define terms, categorize the types of problems addressed by research for universal health coverage, and describe activities in the research cycle (Box 2.1, Box 2.2 and Box 2.3). The intention is to provide a way of thinking about the research process, and to present a classification of research questions and procedures that will be used throughout this report.

Box 2.2.   Classifying research studies: an example

It is helpful to classify the type of research question under investigation, in addition to identifying activities in the research cycle (Box 2.3). One possible classification, devised by the Clinical Research Collaboration in the United Kingdom of Great Britain and Northern Ireland and based partly on the WHO International Classification of Diseases, covers the spectrum of biomedical and health research, from basic to applied (Box 2.1) and across all areas of health and disease. The eight sections below are illustrated with examples of topics included in each; the full classification is available at www.hrcsonline.net (11, 12). Some aspects of section 1, such as normal biological development and functioning, are considered to be outside the scope of research for universal coverage because they do not directly address defined health problems. Section 8 is modified here to distinguish systems (overall structure) and services (delivery within a given system), and also goes beyond health research to embrace the broader concept of research for health (Box 2.1).

1. Underpinning research (basic or fundamental research)

Normal biological development and functioning; psychological and socioeconomic processes; chemical and physical sciences; methodologies and measurements (including disease burden); resources and infrastructure.

2. Etiology (causation)

Biological and endogenous factors; factors relating to the physical environment; psychological, social and economic factors; surveillance and distribution; research design and methodologies.

3. Prevention of disease and conditions, and promotion of well-being

Primary prevention interventions to modify behaviours or promote well-being; interventions to alter physical and biological environmental risks; nutrition and chemoprevention; vaccines.

4. Detection, screening and diagnosis

Discovery and preclinical testing of markers and technologies; evaluation of markers and diagnostic technologies; population screening.

5. Development of treatments and therapeutic interventions

Pharmaceuticals, cellular and gene therapies; medical devices; surgery; radiotherapy; psychological and behavioural interventions; physical and complementary treatments.

6. Evaluation of treatments and therapeutic interventions

Pharmaceuticals; cellular and gene therapies; medical devices; surgery; radiotherapy; psychological and behavioural interventions; physical and complementary treatments.

7. Management of diseases and conditions

Individual care needs; management and decision-making; resources and infrastructure.

8. Health policy and systems research

Organization and delivery of services; health and welfare economics; policy, ethics and research governance; research design and methodologies; resources and infrastructure. The systems and services that benefit health lie both within and beyond the health sector (Box 2.1).

There is no general agreement on ways to classify research. Some would emphasize the methods used and types of questions addressed within the disciplines of economics, epidemiology, statistics and sociology; others would focus on elements of the research cycle in Box 2.3. This particular example is presented because it is also used to organize the case studies in Chapter 3.

Box 2.3. The research cycle: questions, answers, and more questions

Just as this report defines universal health coverage broadly (Chapter 1), it also takes a comprehensive view of the scope of research. This report is concerned with any investigation motivated by the goal of achieving universal coverage – from discovery, through development, to delivery – thereby improving health. Investigations cover all five of the steps depicted in the figure: measuring the size of the health problem; understanding its cause(s); devising solutions; translating the evidence into policy, practice and products; and evaluating effectiveness after implementation. The process of doing research is not linear but cyclical, because each answer brings a new set of questions. This research cycle is often called the "cycle of innovation".

The cycle of research activities, divided into five parts, illustrated here with reference to micronutrient malnutrition

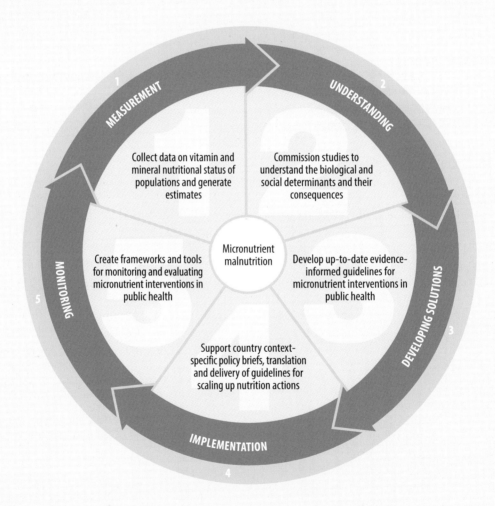

Note: Research begins with measuring and understanding the problem, it proceeds to developing solutions, and then monitors the success of interventions. Monitoring is the source of new questions, so another cycle begins.
Reproduced, by permission of the publisher, from Pena-Rosas et al. (13).

continues ...

... continued

As is made clear in the WHO Strategy on Research for Health, good research needs an enabling environment, which includes mechanisms for agreeing on research priorities, for developing research capacity (staff, funding, institutions), for setting standards in research practice, and for translating the results of research into policy (Chapter 4) (*2*).

The strength of inference that can be made from research studies is dependent partly on the study design, ranging from observational studies (weaker), through cross-sectional, case–control and cohort studies, to randomized controlled trials (stronger) (*14*). To apply the results of a research study in another setting requires causes and effects to be linked in the same way; this is not a matter of study design.

The GRADE (Grading of Recommendations Assessment, Development and Evaluation) system assesses the quality of evidence and the strength of recommendations on the basis of the evidence. It is a transparent and systematic mechanism for judging whether the results of research are robust enough to inform policy (*15*, *16*). At present, GRADE is an effective tool for assessing the value of an intervention studied by a clinical trial, but is less well suited to judging, for example, how easily an intervention can be implemented in a health system, or its suitability with respect to health equity. GRADE has had to be fine-tuned to deal with issues specific to immunization, such as the population-level effects of vaccines, and to the use of data from surveillance systems (*17*). Furthermore, the outputs of GRADE need to be presented in a manner that is accessible to policy-makers. Initiatives such as DECIDE (Developing and Evaluating Communication strategies to support Informed Decisions and practice based on Evidence, http://www.decide-collaboration.eu) are helping to do this. The GRADE working group (www.gradeworkinggroup.org) offers courses and workshops to make best use of the GRADE system.

Creativity everywhere

There is a fear that many of the world's contemporary problems – in health and in other domains – are too complex to understand and too difficult to manage (*18*). This report takes a more positive view. There are undoubtedly many problems that are hard to solve en route to universal health coverage – such as improving the efficiency of health care through the dense network of connections that make up health services. Nevertheless, wherever we look in the world, we find people proposing ingenious solutions to difficult questions about health care (Box 2.4). Creativity is a leitmotif in this report. While creative solutions are to be encouraged, innovations may have unintended adverse consequences and for this reason they require rigorous evaluation.

The stories in Box 2.4 are not isolated examples of applied ingenuity. New ideas are pervasive, as revealed in a 10-country survey of R&D carried out for the 2010 African Innovation Outlook. The study found that there were new concepts behind the development of both products and procedures in private companies of all sizes (*23*).

Drawing on specific examples (Box 2.4) and general surveys, our conclusion is that creativity and imagination are ubiquitous (*23*). The working assumption in this report is that new ideas will throw up potential solutions to health problems, and that innovators will turn some of these proposed solutions into practical applications if they are permitted and encouraged to do so. Some of these practical innovations will be shown by research to be worthy of large-scale implementation.

In the next section we show that the research needed to harness these new ideas is on the rise.

Research ascending

The landmark 1990 report from the Commission on Health Research for Development had a lasting impact by showing that less than 10% of global research spending was targeted at the diseases

Box 2.4. **Problems, ideas, solutions**

....

Innovation in action: mobile phone software developed to monitor fetal movements and heartbeats

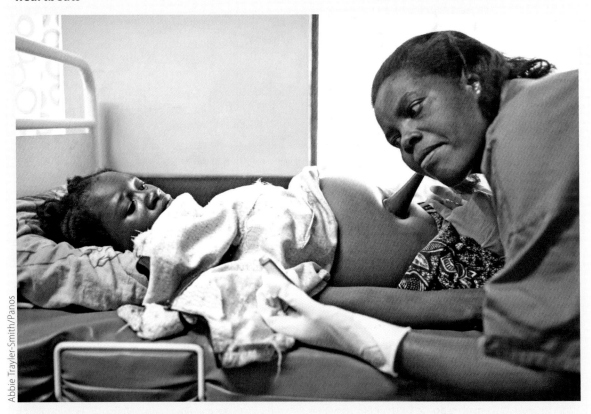

Abbie Trayler-Smith/Panos

Zeinou Abdelyamin from Algeria has been worried that the widespread use of insecticides and rodenticides leaves chemical residues that are harmful to people and domestic animals. In 2012, he won an African Prize for Innovation for carrying out research to formulate nonchemical pesticides that leave no trace in the environment (19).

In the same year, Aaron Tushabe and fellow students at Makerere University, Uganda, wanted to find ways to make pregnancy safer for women who do not have easy access to hospitals (20). They invented a portable scanner to detect anomalies in gestation, such as ectopic pregnancies and abnormal fetal heart beats (see photograph). Cheaper than ultrasound, their hand-held scanner is a funnel-like horn that gives a read-out on the screen of a mobile phone.

Meanwhile in Tamil Nadu, India, Dr V Mohan has created the "self-expanding diabetes clinic" to provide diagnosis and care to people in remote rural areas of India (21). His mobile clinic, housed in a van carrying satellite equipment, visits some of the remotest parts of Tamil Nadu, linking urban doctors to rural patients via community health workers. The van has telemedicine technology to carry out diagnostic tests, such as retinal scans, and transmit the results within seconds to Chennai, even from areas too remote for Internet connectivity. The wider application of these innovations needs to be guided by health technology assessments (22).

The key point, however, is that examples of creativity and innovation can be found everywhere.

Box 2.5.   Milestones in research for health

1990 Report of the independent Commission on Health Research for Development (1)

This report exposed the mismatch between investment in health research in developing countries (5% of all funds) and the burden of disease in these countries, measured as years of life lost through preventable deaths (93%). The mismatch was later characterized by the Global Forum for Health Research as the "10/90 gap" (less than 10% of global spending on research devoted to diseases and conditions that account for 90% of the burden of ill-health) (24). The report recommended that all countries undertake and support essential national health research; that more financial support for research should be obtained through international partnerships; and that an international mechanism should be established to monitor progress.

1996 WHO Ad Hoc Committee on Health Research Relating to Future Intervention Options (25)

The committee identified the best value in health research and suggested that investments be made in four main areas: childhood infectious diseases, microbial threats, noncommunicable diseases and injuries, and weak health systems.

2001 Commission on Macroeconomics and Health (26)

The commissioners made a case for greater investment in health research globally. They called for the establishment of a Global Health Research Fund to support research in areas that primarily affect developing countries, focusing on basic scientific research in health and biomedicine.

2004/5 Ministerial Summit on Health Research in Mexico City (2004) and the associated World Health Assembly Resolution WHA58.34 (2005)

The Ministerial Summit and the World Health Assembly argued for more resources and more research on health systems and health policy to strengthen health systems, supported by the background work of an independent task force convened by WHO (27). They drew attention to the science that is needed to improve health systems, and urged greater efforts to bridge the gap between scientific potential and health improvement. In parallel, WHO launched the *World report on knowledge for better health* (28).

2008 Global Ministerial Forum on Research for Health in Bamako, Mali

The Forum was convened by WHO and five partners with the theme "Strengthening research for health, development and equity". It placed research and innovation within the wider context of research for development. It led to specific recommendations and commitments, culminating in a research plan of action.

2010 and 2012 Global Symposia on Health Systems Research in Montreux and Beijing

These symposia were a response to the heightened interest in health systems research (29). Under the theme of "Science to accelerate universal health coverage" the Montreux symposium called for country ownership in developing the capacity to create stronger health systems. It was proposed that health systems research should become the third pole of medical research, complementing biomedical and clinical research. Beijing followed Montreux with the theme "Inclusion and innovation towards universal health coverage" (www.hsr-symposium.org).

that are responsible for more than 90% of the global burden of ill-health (Box 2.5). Owing to the success of that report, the "10/90 gap" has become short-hand for underinvestment in health research in low-income countries.

More than two decades later, the influential 1990 report and subsequent events (Box 2.5) have made a contribution to the growth of research worldwide. Practically every indicator of research activity has been rising. Systematic

evaluations of the burden of disease have been strongly encouraged since the early 1990s. The reaction, as seen in the scientific literature, has been impressive. There has been a proliferation of published studies of disease burden, carried out at global, regional and national levels (part A of Fig. 2.1) (31). Questions about the scale of a health problem are not always about disease burden (Box 2.2 and Box 2.3), but studies of this kind reflect the upward trend in recognizing and

Fig. 2.1.   Six measures of the growth in research that would support universal health coverage

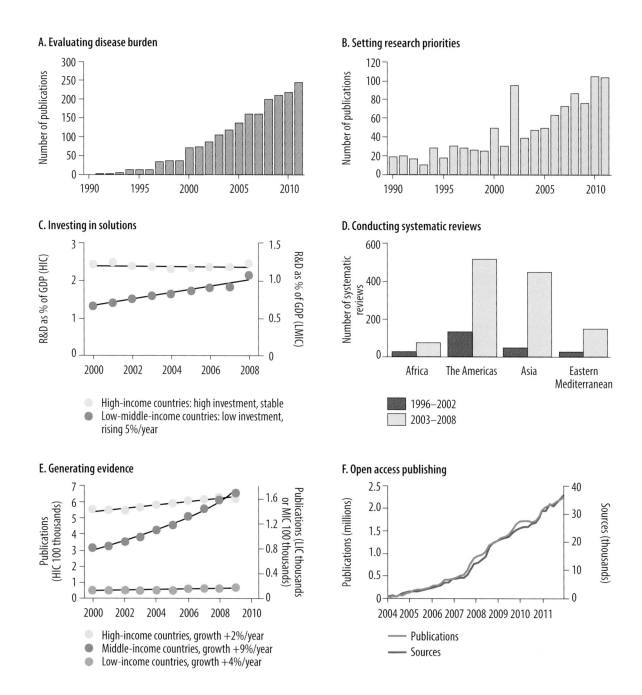

GDP, gross domestic product; HIC, high-income countries; LIM, low-income countries; LMIC, low- and middle-income countries; MIC, middle-income countries; OECD, Organisation for Economic Co-operation and Development; R&D, research and development.

Sources: A and B: www.ncbi.nlm.nih.gov/pubmed; C: OECD; D: Law et al. (*30*); E: The World Bank; F: www.base-search.net.

evaluating health challenges. The improving evidence about major causes of illness and death is a basis for setting research priorities, and published prioritization exercises in this area have increased by a factor of five since 1990 (part B of Fig. 2.1) (*32*). Standard approaches to setting priorities are gaining acceptance worldwide (*33, 34*).

To turn research priorities into research studies requires funding. Investment in R&D has remained static in relation to economic output – i.e. gross domestic product (GDP) – in high-income countries. But in low- and middle-income countries (mostly the latter), domestic investment in R&D has been growing 5% per year faster than economic output (part C of Fig. 2.1). This strong upward trend, which is most visible in China and other eastern Asian countries, emphasizes the importance placed on research by emerging economies (*4*). This trend applies to R&D generally, but it is likely to benefit health too. In the specific area of health policy and systems research, a 2010 survey of 96 research institutions in low-income countries found that funding has been steadily increasing, notably to institutions in sub-Saharan Africa (*35, 36*).

The global financial downturn of the late 2000s slowed the rise in R&D funding for technologies to control "neglected" diseases, which mainly affect low- and middle-income countries. Yet funding was not significantly cut: on aggregate, public funding remained more or less stable between 2009 and 2011 because decreases from philanthropic organizations were offset by greater investment from industry (*37*).

These flattening budgets, set against the persistently large burden of communicable diseases in lower-income countries, have stimulated thinking that is beginning to break the mould of traditional R&D. More products are now being created through partnerships between universities, governments, international organizations and the private sector. In some instances, competition is being replaced by collaboration, and explicit links are being made among the different

organizations involved in discovery, development and deployment of new technologies. The Drugs for Neglected Diseases initiative (DNDi) is working with three pharmaceutical companies to develop a new anthelmintic drug. Together, Health Canada, the Drugs Controller General of India and WHO facilitated the registration and use of a new meningitis A vaccine for Africa (MenAfriVac) in a matter of months (*38*). The evolving structure of research partnerships is helping to prepare the ground for a new generation of medical products and services, such as those oriented to "precision" or "personalized" medicine.

Not only is more research being done in more creative ways, but the process of doing research is also becoming more robust. One illustration is the growth in systematic reviews (of health systems evidence in part D of Fig. 2.1), long-advocated by the Cochrane Collaboration (www.cochrane.org) (*39*). In recent years, the growth in the number of these reviews has been similar in high-income and lower-income countries. There are, however, large differences between individual lower-income countries; comparing the periods 1996–2002 and 2003–2008, the number of systematic reviews of health systems increased 3-fold for Africa and 110-fold for Asia (*30*).

There are now so many systematic reviews of clinical trials that it has become difficult to track and assimilate the huge volume of information. The surfeit of data has led to a plea to devise more efficient ways of keeping up with the evidence (*40*).

More research is generating more evidence to guide policy and practice (part E of Fig. 2.1). On the African continent, research productivity, measured by publications in 19 countries (dominated by Egypt and South Africa), grew at an average rate of 5.3% per year between 1990 and 2009, but that growth was far quicker during the final five years of this period (26% per year). Research productivity in Africa, by African scientists, has been stimulated by concern about HIV/AIDS, tuberculosis and malaria, and is linked to the

Fig. 2.2. **The share of internationally co-authored science and engineering articles worldwide, by country, 2000 and 2010**

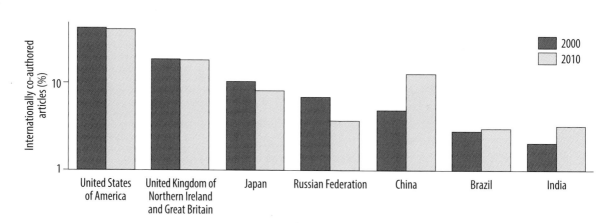

Note: The USA and United Kingdom had high but stable levels of co-authorship; researchers based in the USA were co-authors of 43% of the total number of internationally co-authored articles in 2010. The share of co-authorships in Brazil and India has been low and is growing slowly; in China they have been low but are growing quickly (*4*).

establishment of national public health training institutions (*41*). A 26-country survey of health systems research found that the number of investigations increased over the past decade, and that decisions about health policy were based on evidence in about two thirds of the sampled countries (Chapter 4) (*42*). Health policy and systems research is beginning to flourish although, in the view of some commentators, it is not yet a fully coherent enterprise (*29, 43*).

More research is being published as a result of international collaboration. While it is still the case that a minority of studies are led by scientists from low- and middle-income countries, these researchers are increasingly working in international partnerships. China is the outstanding example: the global share of co-authorships held by Chinese researchers increased from 5% in 2000 to 13% in 2010 (Fig. 2.2). Among the seven countries for which data are shown in Fig. 2.2 (Brazil, China, India, Japan, Russian Federation, United Kingdom of Great Britain and Northern Ireland, United States of America), China enjoyed the biggest increase in co-authorships in both absolute and relative terms.

As the number of publications grows, more of the results are becoming freely available through "open access" arrangements that give unrestricted access via the Internet to peer-reviewed journal articles (part F of Fig. 2.1) (*44*). In the same spirit, the HINARI Access to Research in Health Programme was created in 2001 to provide wider access to the world's biomedical literature, although the scheme requires affiliation to a registered institution. HINARI is now one of the four programmes comprising Research4Life (along with Research in Agriculture, Research in the Environment, and Research for Development and Innovation). By the tenth anniversary of this programme, Research4Life had provided researchers at 6000 institutions in 100 developing countries with free or low-cost access to 9000 journals on health, agriculture, environment and technology (*45*).

The scope of research for health is widening too. As the world contemplates the transition from the MDGs to a post-2015 development agenda, greater emphasis is being placed on research carried out in all sectors that affect health (the "health in all sectors" approach) – e.g.

Box 2.6.   Environmental health research, "health in all", and universal health coverage

Roughly one quarter of the global burden of disease can be attributed to modifiable environmental risk factors (*46*). This is an approximate estimate because our understanding of the links between our environment and health, and of how to mitigate the risks to health, is far from complete. Further research therefore needs to cover a wide range of investigations from the evaluation of risks associated with environmental exposures, through mechanisms for prevention, to ways of incorporating these measures into the delivery of services (Box 2.2). The solutions that reduce environmental health risks will come from both within the health sector and beyond it.

Environmental risk factors are physical, chemical and biological hazards that directly affect health, and also factors that exacerbate unhealthy behaviours (e.g. physical inactivity). Environmental risk factors include unsafe drinking-water and poor sanitation and hygiene, which are the sources of infections that cause diarrhoeal diseases. According to one global assessment of risk factors for ill-health, unimproved water and poor sanitation have fallen in importance in the ranking of risk factors but nevertheless accounted for 0.9% of all years of healthy life lost (i.e. disability-adjusted life-years, or DALYs) in 2010 (*47*). Environmental risk factors include indoor air pollution, largely from the use of solid fuels in households, and outdoor air pollution, which facilitate and exacerbate lower respiratory infections. Household air pollution was a leading risk factor for ill-health in sub-Saharan Africa and southern Asia in 2010 (*47*). Risk factors include injuries arising from hazards in the workplace, from radiation and from industrial accidents. They also contribute to the transmission of vector-borne diseases: malaria is associated with policies and practices on land use, deforestation, water resource management, settlement siting and house design.

Universal health coverage explicitly includes preventive measures (Chapter 1) where their primary purpose is to improve health, and yet the opportunities to prevent ill-health have often been overlooked, both within and outside the health sector. The "Health in the Green Economy" project provides numerous examples of research that identify environmental health benefits that come from mitigating climate change. These illustrate how policies whose primary objective are not to achieve universal health coverage but rather to confront environmental threats can yield major health co-benefits. The health system can play an important role in advocating for such policies, which are complementary to effort to promote universal health coverage. Two examples of sectors in which research has demonstrated health co-benefits are urban transport and housing:

- **Urban transport**. More investment in public transport (buses and trains), along with networks for cyclists and pedestrians, can lower urban air pollution, encourage physical activity, lessen traffic injuries, and reduce the costs of mobility for poor and vulnerable groups (*48*). Studies of urban commuters in Shanghai and Copenhagen, for instance, have shown that cyclists have 30% lower mortality rates, on average, than other commuters (*49*).
- **Housing and home energy systems**. Better home insulation, plus energy-efficient, smoke-free heating and cooking systems and indoor ventilation, can reduce respiratory diseases, including asthma, pneumonia and tuberculosis, as well as reducing vulnerability to extremes of heat and cold. Large savings in health costs from asthma and other respiratory illness were observed in follow-up studies of home insulation in low-income homes in New Zealand. The promise of immediate health gains helped drive large-scale government investments in home improvements in New Zealand. To these short-term gains must be added the economic value of carbon savings that will be realized in future (*50*).

Economic research can help define where technological development yields the greatest health benefits for the least cost, driving a virtuous circle of "healthwise" green investments. For instance, improved stove and fuel technologies used in the poorest households in Africa or Latin America are likely to be cheap and effective, but the best available technologies have yet to be evaluated. Shifting away from diesel fuel for transport and energy not only reduces exposures to harmful carcinogens but also cuts climate-changing black carbon.

Following the Rio +20 United Nations Conference on Sustainable Development, a dialogue among governments, United Nations agencies, and civil society will lead to a new set of development goals (*51, 52*). This is an opportunity to highlight the connections between policies that affect health via different sectors of the economy – not just environment and health, but also agriculture, education, finance, social policy and health. Coupled with this is the need for appropriate data and indicators (see also Box 1.2). The research underpinning "health in all sectors" is, in the broad definition of this report, research for universal health coverage.

agriculture, education, environment and finance (Box 2.6) (*51*).

Finally, there is an increasingly energetic debate about how to answer questions about public health; this is a sign of a healthy research environment (*53*). One area of discussion concerns the study of health systems. Victora and co-workers have argued that randomized controlled trials, while essential for measuring the efficacy of clinical interventions, are unsuitable for public health interventions in which there are numerous steps between the possible cause under investigation and the final effect, and where one or more of these steps depends on local circumstances (*54*). By contrast, Banerjee & Duflo have championed the use of randomized controlled trials rigorously to test ideas about how to achieve higher coverage of interventions that depend on human behaviour (*55, 56*). The discussion points to a fundamental truth about randomized controlled trials: a controlled experiment yields rigorous results under the conditions of that experiment. However, whether the result applies beyond the experiment depends on the nature of the system under investigation. In terms of consistency from one setting to another, human biochemical pathways, for instance, are likely to be more consistent than some human behaviours (see also Chapter 3).

None of the rising indicators of research activity, in any setting, is a guarantee of interventions that will help to reach universal health coverage. However, universal coverage cannot be achieved without technology, systems and services, and research is the mechanism by which the hardware and software are created.

Growing unevenly

Research is on the rise, and the results are delivering benefits for health worldwide. However, the process of doing research – setting research priorities, building capacity, formulating and adopting standards of practice, and translating results into policy (Box 2.3) – is certainly not of a uniformly high standard. In many settings, research practice falls well short of the global ideal. But by defining the achievements, and not merely the defects, we shall be in a stronger position to exploit the potential that research offers.

Any survey of the growing strengths in research also exposes the residual weaknesses. In view of the environment needed to carry out research and the sequence of steps in the research cycle, research programmes around the world can be strengthened in a number of areas (Box 2.3).

The number and proportion of older people are increasing in populations around the world, and yet some prominent causes of illness among the elderly are poorly defined. In countries in the Americas Region, for instance, there is a huge variation in reported death rates from Parkinson disease. This variation is more likely to be explained by diagnostic and reporting inaccuracies than by real differences in death rates, but the truth about Parkinson disease will be determined only by systematic investigation. In general, data defining the frequency and health consequences of mental and nervous system disorders are poor (*57*). Much better information is needed to determine how many people are at risk of these disorders or are eligible for treatment, and who they are and where they live (*58–60*).

The growth in research effort, addressing many different questions in a wide variety of settings, is bound to be uneven. There are now hundreds of published studies that focus on specific diseases and conditions – across a range of communicable and noncommunicable diseases and injuries (*61*). In contrast, there are relatively few studies that attempt to set research priorities, across all aspects of health, from the perspective of national governments (Chapter 4) (*62, 63*). This is because few appraisals of research needs have been initiated by national governments, even though such appraisals are a vital part of planning for universal health coverage.

National research portfolios are mostly unplanned, but they may not be wholly

Fig. 2.3.   **Private- and public-sector investment in R&D, classified as basic, applied and experimental development research, for six African countries ranked in ascending order of gross national income (left to right)**

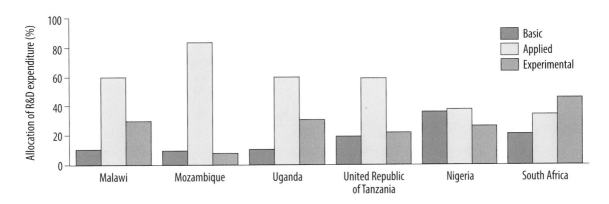

R&D, research and development.
Note: For definitions of types of research, see Box 2.1. The four poorest countries focused on applied research. The two wealthiest, Nigeria and South Africa, had a more balanced portfolio (35).

unbalanced. The 2010 African Innovation Outlook found that four lower-income countries focused on applied research, whereas two richer ones spread resources more evenly across basic, applied and experimental studies (Fig. 2.3). A more systematic look at research in these countries might find that the balance is right, or that it should change. The point is that some questions about universal health coverage have answers that are widely applicable (e.g. the efficacy of a drug against a defined medical condition), but others need local solutions (e.g. how best to deliver the drug to all who need it) (64, 65). For this reason, all nations need to become producers of research as well as consumers of it. Local expertise and local processes, initiatives and institutions should be valued rather than bypassed (64, 66).

Raising funds is one of the challenges in turning research priorities into research studies, and the constraints on fundraising come in various forms. At the level of national wealth, gross national income (GNI) is an empirical measure of research potential. The data in Fig. 2.4 show how research productivity increases disproportionately with national wealth. As a rule of

thumb, for every 10-fold increase in GNI per person, the number of scientific publications per person increases by a factor of about 50 at best (Fig. 2.4, diagonal line). This disproportionate increase also holds for other measures of research output such as the number of researchers and the number of patents per head of population.

These data also show that while some countries exploit the empirical maximum (lying close to the diagonal line in Fig. 2.4), many do not (thus falling below the diagonal line) (67). Some of the countries that fall below the line are nations with small populations (< 20 million), who may choose not to invest in research, but not all underinvestors are small nations. By comparing countries, it can be said that there is much unfulfilled research potential, given national wealth. Thus greater wealth appears to open up the potential for research, but other factors are needed to fulfil that potential. While those factors need to be understood, it is clear that nations and their governments have a choice about how much to invest in research and about what research topics should be given priority.

Fig. 2.4. **National wealth facilitates, but does not guarantee, national research productivity**

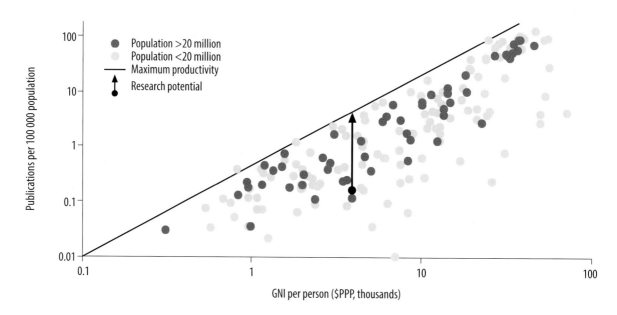

PPP, purchasing power parity.

Note: For every 10-fold increase in gross national income (GNI) per person, the number of scientific publications (per person) increases by a factor of about 50 at best (actually by $10^{5/3} = 46$, diagonal line).

Each point represents a single country. While some countries exploit maximum productivity, lying close to the diagonal line, many lie well below it, indicating that there is unfulfilled research potential, given their national wealth. Some of these countries have smaller populations (< 20 million, blue circles), but not all. The unfulfilled potential for research in one large country (Philippines) is indicated by the vertical arrow.

Source: The World Bank, latest data 2009.

Private companies engaged in R&D in low-income countries frequently cite lack of funding and the shortage of skilled researchers as major barriers to innovation (*35*). The shortage of trained researchers emerges as a general constraint in R&D, but it is also found in specific areas such as health systems research (*36*). A disincentive for private technological research is the domination of R&D by a few established enterprises, with apparently few opportunities for newcomers. A further impediment in low-income countries is poor access to information on technologies and markets for the products (*35*).

There are also disincentives linked to intellectual property rights. The protection of new ideas as intellectual property encourages the development of new medicines and technologies.

However, the products are sold to people who can afford them, often excluding those in greatest need. Both free knowledge (as a public good) and highly restricted knowledge (limited by its proprietary nature) can be obstacles to improving health; the former may discourage innovation and the latter may limit access to the products of innovation. "Market failures" are the enemy of universal health coverage, and the facts about market failure in different settings present some critical questions for research (Box 2.7) (*71, 72*). In this context, WHO expert working groups have sought to promote R&D in ways whereby market failures are rectified by the production of public goods (*67, 68, 73*).

The problem of low investment in research within low-income countries (Fig. 2.4) is amplified

Box 2.7.   The Global Strategy and Plan of Action on Public Health, Innovation and Intellectual Property

Born out of concern among low- and middle-income countries about inequitable access to the products of research, the Commission on Intellectual Property Rights, Innovation and Public Health was established to promote innovation and access to medicines. The work of the Commission led to the Global Strategy and Plan of Action on Public Health, Innovation and Intellectual Property (GSPA-PHI), which was approved by the World Health Assembly in 2009 (*68*).

The GSPA-PHI consists of eight elements that aim to promote innovation, build capacity, improve access and mobilize resources. The eight elements are:

1. prioritize research and development needs;

2. promote research and development;

3. build and improve innovative capacity;

4. transfer of technology;

5. apply and manage intellectual property to contribute to innovation and promote public health;

6. improve delivery and access;

7. promote sustainable financing; and

8. establish monitoring and reporting systems.

Work is under way in several areas related to GSPA-PHI, such as the local production of medical products and technology transfer (element 4), building capacity in the management and use of intellectual property in favour of public health (element 5), reporting on models for sustainable financing and better coordination of research and development (element 7) through WHO expert working groups; and the establishment of monitoring and reporting systems (element 8), such as research observatories (Chapter 4) (*69, 70*).

Effective implementation of the GSPA-PHI depends on the robustness of the national health research system in each country. Over time, monitoring and evaluation will reveal whether the GSPA-PHI leads to increased innovation and more affordable and equitable access to the benefits and products of research, especially in low- and middle-income countries.

by a bias against the type of research that would benefit these countries. In total, more than US$ 100 billion is spent globally on health research each year (*71*). About half of this is in the private sector, mainly in the pharmaceutical and biotechnology industries, and the products of this research are directed mainly at markets in high-income countries (*71, 74*). Drug development is a case in point: only 21 of 1556 (1.3%) new drugs developed over the 30-year period from 1975 to 2004 were for diseases not found in high-income countries (*75*). Despite the persistently high burden of infection in low- and middle-income countries, and the spread of antibiotic resistance, the development of new antibiotics lies in the hands of just a few major

pharmaceutical companies (*76*). More positively, however, methods of preventing and treating noncommunicable diseases, largely developed in richer countries, should help to address the growing burden of these diseases in poorer countries.

In addition, financial investment in basic research and in discovery and development (pharmaceuticals and biotechnology) dwarfs investment in delivery. One survey of 140 health research funders globally found that most research is directed at developing new health technologies rather than at making better use of existing ones (*77*).

For neglected diseases, an imbalance arises because investment favours some infections and diseases over others. Funding for R&D is predominantly for HIV/AIDS, tuberculosis and malaria, with relatively little for some other major causes of ill-health such as dengue, diarrhoeal diseases and helminth infections (*37*).

With respect to delivering health care, research into health services and systems gets relatively little support and tends to be narrowly focused. This is true both in low- and high-income countries. In the United Kingdom in 2006, health services research (included in category 8 in Box 2.2) received between 0.4% and 1.6% of all research funds allocated by four major funding bodies (*78*). Although the United Kingdom's National Institute for Health Research is helping to boost funding for research on health services and systems, these data show that some important funding agencies give this area low priority. An observation repeatedly made in a variety of settings is that too little attention is given to translating existing knowledge about products and processes into policy and practice (*79–81*). Furthermore, the contribution of the social sciences to research in this area, going beyond clinical studies and epidemiology, is commonly undervalued (*2*).

Even when research funds are provided as official development assistance to low-income countries, they are not seen as uniformly beneficial. In the opinion of some African researchers, external aid undermines efforts to convince African governments to spend more money on research (*82*). In the domain of health policy and systems research, a drawback of external funding is that it tends to focus on operational matters, such as how to scale up priority services. On the one hand, external donations to carry out operational and translational research satisfy a pressing need. Yet on the other hand, less attention is given to deeper, structural questions about the functioning of health services – questions that ask, for example, how to promote accountability in service delivery or how to engage local stakeholders (*2*). Observations of this kind highlight a particular challenge in funding research, which is to ensure that the priorities of international donors are aligned with those of national health services, in keeping with the Paris Declaration on Aid Effectiveness (2005), the Accra Agenda for Action (2008) (*83*), and the wider goal of effective development as promoted by the Busan Global Partnership for Effective Development Cooperation (*84*).

In assessing the strengths and weaknesses of research, the virtues of tracking research investments, practices and applications quickly become clear. Such data are absent or incomplete for many countries. To build most effectively on existing foundations, all nations should take a systematic approach to the mapping, monitoring and evaluation of research (*85, 86*).

The value of health research

Adding to the impetus to do more research is a growing body of evidence on the returns on investment, albeit mostly from high-income countries. Notwithstanding some contentious methodological issues – such as how to value health gained, whether in terms of increased survival or improved quality of life – there is mounting quantitative proof of the benefits of research to health, society and the economy (*87*).

Exceptional returns, a report prepared for Funding First in the USA, calculated large gains from reductions in mortality, especially due to cardiovascular disease (*88*). Based on a high figure for the value of a life, the monetary returns from investments in research were valued at US$ 1.5 trillion annually between 1970 and 1990, one third of which was attributed to research into new drugs and treatment protocols. For research on cardiovascular disease, the returns on investment were approximately 20 times the annual expenditure. Access Economics carried out a similar study in Australia, finding that every dollar invested in Australian health research and development yielded, on average, AUS$ 2.17 (approximately US$ 2.27) in health benefits. This rate of return was surpassed only in the mining and retail sectors (*89*).

The benefits of randomized controlled trials of drug treatments and clinical procedures, funded by the National Institute of Neurological Disorders and Stroke in the USA, have also been evaluated in monetary terms (*90*). The assessment included 28 trials carried out at a total cost of US$ 335 million. By valuing a quality-adjusted life year (QALY) as the same as gross domestic product (GDP) per capita, the projected net benefit to society after 10 years was US$ 15·2 billion, indicating a yearly return on investment of 46%.

In the United Kingdom, a study of cardiovascular disease and mental health research separated the value of the gain to health (QALYs valued at £25 000, as used in the United Kingdom's National Health Service) from the gain to the economy (GDP), with the latter resulting from the wider economic effects of public and charitable research spending, including the stimulus to privately-funded research (*87*). The yearly rate of return with respect to the health gain was 9% for cardiovascular disease research, and 7% for mental health research. The yearly rate of return in terms of GDP was 30% for all medical research in the United Kingdom. Putting these together gave a total yearly rate of return of 39% for cardiovascular disease and mental health research in the United Kingdom over a period of 17 years.

Not all the benefits of research can be, or should be, measured in monetary terms (*91*). To capture the diversity of benefits from research, the Payback Framework evaluates outcomes under five headings: knowledge, benefits to future research and research use, benefits from informing policy and product development, health and health sector benefits, and economic benefits (*91–96*). This model of assessment has logical appeal because, while acknowledging complexities and feedback loops, it tracks the evolution of a research idea from its inception, through the research process into dissemination, and on to its impact on health, society and the economy (*92, 97*). It parallels the research cycle depicted in Box 2.3.

The Payback Framework has been used in Ireland, for instance, to assess the benefits of a pilot project on the early detection of psychosis (*98*). The study described how the early intervention services, contributing to the Irish mental health service, could reduce the duration of untreated psychosis, the severity of symptoms, suicidal behaviour and the rate of relapse and subsequent hospitalization. The study suggested that early detection reduces the cost of treatment, saves lives, and is highly regarded both by those who use the service and by their families.

Besides evaluating the returns on research, one should also consider the source of the initial investment and how it affects access to the products of the research. For instance, public-sector research institutions in the USA do more applied research than has sometimes been thought. In one domain, they contributed to the discovery of 9–21% of all drugs involved in new-drug applications that were approved between 1990 and 2007 (*99*). Publicly funded research in the USA also tends to discover drugs that are expected to have disproportionately large clinical effects.

A conspicuous feature of studies that assess the economic value of research is that, according to one review, none have yet been carried out in low- and middle-income countries. A key concern, therefore, is how far such countries can rely on medical research carried out elsewhere (*91*).

Conclusions: building on the foundations

Research for universal health coverage is not a luxury; rather, it is fundamental to the discovery, development and delivery of interventions that people need to maintain good health (*100*). If "the best days for public health are ahead of us" it will be, in part, because the best days for health research also lie ahead (*101*).

The 1990 report of the Commission on Health Research for Development has a legacy (*102*). The report generated a wide appreciation of the shortfall in research investment and of the fragility of health research in low- and middle-income countries. More than 20 years later, it is clear that research for health is on the rise worldwide. Health problems are better defined than they were two decades ago. There are more funds and greater research capacity to address key questions about health. Investigations are increasingly following best practice in design, ethics and the reporting of results. There are more research institutions and networks, and there is more national and international collaboration, "south to south" as well as "north to south" (*103*). The review of the research landscape in this chapter is not yet a story of research potential fulfilled but it shows the strengthening foundations on which better research programmes can now be built.

Creativity and imagination are central to the research enterprise. A premise of this report is that, wherever people have health problems, new ideas will be proposed to help solve them. The constraints are in the means of turning these ideas into dependable, practical applications. Even research of the highest quality does not automatically translate into better health if the findings are not implemented.

To better understand the task ahead, there is a need systematically to assess the strengths and weaknesses of research for health, country by country, worldwide. When public money is being spent on research, there should be mechanisms for debating research priorities, for developing the capacity to carry out research, for setting standards, and for translating the results into policy and practice. In judging the priorities for spending, there should be a consensus on the balance of activities related to the research cycle: measuring the size of the health problem; understanding its cause; devising solutions; translating the evidence into policy, practice and products; and evaluating the effectiveness of interventions after implementation. Further, for any problem studied in any given setting, there should be discussion on the methods of investigation, the significance of the findings, and the inferences to be drawn from them.

The means of creating a healthy research environment and of judging its performance are described in greater detail in Chapter 4. However, before considering how to establish effective research programmes, Chapter 3 shows how research can address some of the big questions about universal health coverage in order to provide credible answers to inform policy and practice. ■

References

1. Commission on Health Research for Development. *Health research - essential link to equity in development*. Oxford, Oxford University Press, 1990.
2. *WHO strategy on research for health*. Geneva, World Health Organization, 2012. (http://www.who.int/phi/WHO_Strategy_on_research_for_health.pdf, accessed 23 April 2013).
3. *Research assessment exercise. Guidance on submissions*. London, Higher Education Funding Council for England, 2005.
4. National Science Board. *Science and engineering indicators 2012*. Arlington, VA, National Science Foundation, 2012.
5. Humphreys K, Piot P. Scientific evidence alone is not sufficient basis for health policy. *BMJ (Clinical Research Ed.)*, 2012,344:e1316. doi: http://dx.doi.org/10.1136/bmj.e1316 PMID:22371864
6. *Glossary of statistical terms*. Paris, Organisation for Economic Co-operation and Development, 2012. (stats.oecd.org/glossary/search.asp, accessed 14 March 2013).
7. Zachariah R et al. Is operational research delivering the goods? The journey to success in low-income countries. *The Lancet Infectious Diseases*, 2012,12:415-421. doi: http://dx.doi.org/10.1016/S1473-3099(11)70309-7 PMID:22326018
8. Lobb R, Colditz GA. Implementation science and its application to population health. *Annual Review of Public Health*, 2013,34:235-251. doi: http://dx.doi.org/10.1146/annurev-publhealth-031912-114444 PMID:23297655

9.   *Translational research*. Seattle, Institute of Translational Health Sciences, 2012 (www.iths.org, accessed 14 March 2013).

10. Alliance for Health Policy and Systems Research. What is HPSR? Overview (web page). Geneva, World Health Organization, 2011.

11. *Health research classification system*. London, UK Clinical Research Collaboration, 2009.

12. *Health research classification systems: current approaches and future recommendations*. Strasbourg, European Science Foundation, 2011.

13. Pena-Rosas JP et al. Translating research into action: WHO evidence-informed guidelines for safe and effective micronutrient interventions. *The Journal of Nutrition*, 2012,142:197S-204S. doi: http://dx.doi.org/10.3945/jn.111.138834 PMID:22113868

14. Bonita R, Beaglehole R, Kjellström T. *Basic epidemiology*, 2nd ed. Geneva, World Health Organization, 2006.

15. Guyatt GH et al. GRADE: an emerging consensus on rating quality of evidence and strength of recommendations. *BMJ (Clinical Research Ed.)*, 2008,336:924-926. doi: http://dx.doi.org/10.1136/bmj.39489.470347.AD PMID:18436948

16. *WHO handbook for guideline development*. Geneva, World Health Organization, 2012.

17. Duclos P et al. Developing evidence-based immunization recommendations and GRADE. *Vaccine*, 2012,31:12-19. doi: http://dx.doi.org/10.1016/j.vaccine.2012.02.041 PMID:22391401

18. Homer-Dixon T. *The ingenuity gap*. London, Vintage Books, 2001.

19. *Innovation Prize for Africa*. Addis Ababa, United Nations Economic Commission for Africa and the African Innovation Foundation, 2011 (www.innovationprizeforafrica.org, accessed 14 March 2013).

20. Nakkazi E. *Students develop software to monitor unborn babies*. AllAfrica, 2012. (allafrica.com/stories/201205240064.html, accessed 14 March 2013).

21. Dr. Mohan's Diabetes Specialities Centre (web site). Chennai, Dr. Mohan's, 2012. (www.drmohansdiabetes.com, accessed 14 March 2013).

22. *Priority-setting in health: building institutions for smarter public spending*. Washington, DC, Center for Global Development, 2012.

23. Omachonu VK, Einspruch NG. Innovation in healthcare delivery systems: a conceptual framework. *The Innovation Journal: The Public Sector Innovation Journal*, 2010,15(1).

24. *The 10/90 report on health research 2000*. Geneva, Global Forum for Health Research, 2000.

25. *Investing in health research and development. Report of the Ad Hoc Committee on Health Research Relating to Future Intervention Options*. Geneva, World Health Organization, 1996.

26. *Macroeconomics and health: Investing in health for economic development. Report of the Commission on Macroeconomics and Health*. Geneva, World Health Organization, 2001.

27. Task Force on Health Systems Research. Informed choices for attaining the Millennium Development Goals: towards an international cooperative agenda for health-systems research. *Lancet*, 2004,364:997-1003. doi: http://dx.doi.org/10.1016/S0140-6736(04)17026-8 PMID:15364193

28. *World report on knowledge for better health – strengthening health systems*. Geneva, World Health Organization, 2004.

29. Hafner T, Shiffman J. The emergence of global attention to health systems strengthening. *Health Policy and Planning*, 2013,28:41-50. doi: http://dx.doi.org/10.1093/heapol/czs023 PMID:22407017

30. Law T et al. Climate for evidence-informed health systems: a profile of systematic review production in 41 low- and middle-income countries, 1996–2008. *Journal of Health Services Research & Policy*, 2012,17:4-10. doi: http://dx.doi.org/10.1258/jhsrp.2011.010109 PMID:21967823

31. Murray CJ et al. GBD 2010: a multi-investigator collaboration for global comparative descriptive epidemiology. *Lancet*, 2012,380:2055-2058. doi: http://dx.doi.org/10.1016/S0140-6736(12)62134-5 PMID:23245598

32. Youngkong S, Kapiriri L, Baltussen R. Setting priorities for health interventions in developing countries: a review of empirical studies. *Tropical Medicine & International Health*, 2009,14:930-939. doi: http://dx.doi.org/10.1111/j.1365-3156.2009.02311.x PMID:19563479

33. Viergever RF et al. A checklist for health research priority setting: nine common themes of good practice. *Health Research Policy and Systems*, 2010,8:36. PMID:21159163

34. Rudan I. Global health research priorities: mobilizing the developing world. *Public Health*, 2012,126:237-240. doi: http://dx.doi.org/10.1016/j.puhe.2011.12.001 PMID:22325672

35. AU-NEPAD (African Union – New Partnership for Africa's Development). *African innovation outlook 2010*. Pretoria, AU-NEPAD, 2010.

36. Adam T et al. Trends in health policy and systems research over the past decade: still too little capacity in low-income countries. *PLoS ONE*, 2011,6:e27263. doi: http://dx.doi.org/10.1371/journal.pone.0027263 PMID:22132094

37. *Neglected disease research and development: a five year review*. Sydney, Policy Cures, 2012.

38. Mundel T. Global health needs to fill the innovation gap. *Nature Medicine*, 2012,18:1735. doi: http://dx.doi.org/10.1038/nm1212-1735 PMID:23223055

39. Chalmers I, Hedges LV, Cooper H. A brief history of research synthesis. *Evaluation & the Health Professions*, 2002,25:12-37. doi: http://dx.doi.org/10.1177/0163278702025001003 PMID:11868442

40. Bastian H, Glasziou P, Chalmers I. Seventy-five trials and eleven systematic reviews a day: how will we ever keep up? *PLoS Medicine*, 2010,7:e1000326. doi: http://dx.doi.org/10.1371/journal.pmed.1000326 PMID:20877712

41. Nachega JB et al. Current status and future prospects of epidemiology and public health training and research in the WHO African region. *International Journal of Epidemiology*, 2012,41:1829-1846. doi: http://dx.doi.org/10.1093/ije/dys189 PMID:23283719

42. Decoster K, Appelmans A, Hill P. *A health systems research mapping exercise in 26 low- and middle-income countries: narratives from health systems researchers, policy brokers and policy-makers.* (Background paper commissioned by the Alliance for Health Policy and Systems Research to develop the WHO Health Systems Research Strategy). Geneva, Alliance for Health Policy and Systems Research, World Health Organization, 2012.

43. Sheikh K et al. Building the field of health policy and systems research: framing the questions. *PLoS Medicine*, 2011,8:e1001073. doi: http://dx.doi.org/10.1371/journal.pmed.1001073 PMID:21857809

44. *Global Open Access Portal*. Paris, United Nations Educational, Scientific and Cultural Organization, 2012. (http://www.unesco.org/new/en/communication-and-information/portals-and-platforms/goap/, accessed 14 March 2012).

45. *Making a difference*. Geneva, Research4Life, 2011.

46. Prüss-Üstün A, Corvalán C. *Preventing disease through healthy environments. Towards an estimate of the environmental burden of disease*. Geneva, World Health Organization, 2006.

47. Lim SS et al. A comparative risk assessment of burden of disease and injury attributable to 67 risk factors and risk factor clusters in 21 regions, 1990–2010: a systematic analysis for the Global Burden of Disease Study 2010. *Lancet*, 2012,380:2224-2260. doi: http://dx.doi.org/10.1016/S0140-6736(12)61766-8 PMID:23245609

48. Dora C et al. *Urban transport and health. Module 5g. Sustainable transport: a sourcebook for policy-makers in developing cities*. Eschborn, Deutsche Gesellschaft für Internationale Zusammenarbeit, and Geneva, World Health Organization, 2011.

49. *Health in the green economy: health co-benefits of climate change mitigation – transport sector*. Geneva, World Health Organization, 2011.

50. *Health in the green economy: health co-benefits of climate change mitigation – housing sector*. Geneva, World Health Organization, 2011.

51. *Sustainable development goals*. New York, United Nations, 2013. (sustainabledevelopment.un.org, accessed 14 March 2013).

52. Haines A et al. From the Earth Summit to Rio+20: integration of health and sustainable development. *Lancet*, 2012,379:2189-2197. doi: http://dx.doi.org/10.1016/S0140-6736(12)60779-X PMID:22682465

53. Gilbert N. International aid projects come under the microscope. *Nature*, 2013,493:462-463. doi: http://dx.doi.org/10.1038/493462a PMID:23344337

54. Victora CG, Habicht JP, Bryce J. Evidence-based public health: moving beyond randomized trials. *American Journal of Public Health*, 2004,94:400-405. doi: http://dx.doi.org/10.2105/AJPH.94.3.400 PMID:14998803

55. Banerjee AV, Duflos E. *Poor economics*. New York, NY, PublicAffairs, 2011.

56. Duflo E. Rigorous evaluation of human behavior. *Science*, 2012,336:1398. doi: http://dx.doi.org/10.1126/science.1224965 PMID:22700919

57. Eaton WW et al. The burden of mental disorders. *Epidemiologic Reviews*, 2008,30:1-14. doi: http://dx.doi.org/10.1093/epirev/mxn011 PMID:18806255

58. Yasamy MT et al. Responsible governance for mental health research in low resource countries. *PLoS Medicine*, 2011,8:e1001126. doi: http://dx.doi.org/10.1371/journal.pmed.1001126 PMID:22131909

59. Tol WA et al. Research priorities for mental health and psychosocial support in humanitarian settings. *PLoS Medicine*, 2011,8:e1001096. doi: http://dx.doi.org/10.1371/journal.pmed.1001096 PMID:21949644

60. *Challenges and priorities for global mental health research in low- and middle-income countries*. London, Academy of Medical Sciences, 2008.

61. Pang T, Terry RF. PLoS Medicine editors. WHO/PLoS collection "No health without research": a call for papers. *PLoS Medicine*, 2011,8:e1001008. doi: http://dx.doi.org/10.1371/journal.pmed.1001008

62. Tomlinson M et al. A review of selected research priority setting processes at national level in low and middle income countries: towards fair and legitimate priority setting. *Health Research Policy and Systems*, 2011,9:19. doi: http://dx.doi.org/10.1186/1478-4505-9-19 PMID:21575144

63. Alger J et al. Sistemas nacionales de investigación para la salud en América Latina: una revisión de 14 países [National health research systems in Latin America: a 14-country review]. *Revista Panamericana de Salud Pública*, 2009,26:447-457. PMID:20107697

64. Victora CG et al. Achieving universal coverage with health interventions. *Lancet*, 2004,364:1541-1548. doi: http://dx.doi.org/10.1016/S0140-6736(04)17279-6 PMID:15500901

65. *Knowledge translation on ageing and health: a framework for policy development*. Geneva, World Health Organization, 2012.

66. *Planning, monitoring and evaluation framework for capacity strengthening in health research* (ESSENCE Good practice document series. Document TDR/ESSENCE/11.1). Geneva, World Health Organization, 2011.

67. McKee M, Stuckler D, Basu S. Where there is no health research: what can be done to fill the global gaps in health research? *PLoS Medicine*, 2012,9:e1001209. doi: http://dx.doi.org/10.1371/journal.pmed.1001209 PMID:22545025

68. *Global strategy and plan of action on public health, innovation and intellectual property*. Geneva, World Health Organization, 2011.

69. *Research and development to meet health needs in developing countries: strengthening global financing and coordination. Report of the Consultative Expert Working Group on Research and Development: Financing and Coordination*. Geneva, World Health Organization, 2012.

70. *Research and development – coordination and financing. Report of the Expert Working Group*. Geneva, World Health Organization, 2010.

71. *Public health, innovation and intellectual property rights: report of the Commission on Intellectual Property Rights, Innovation and Public Health*. Geneva, World Health Organization, 2006.

72. *Promoting access to medical technologies and innovation: intersections between public health, intellectual property and trade*. Geneva, World Health Organization, World Intellectual Property Organization and World Trade Organization, 2013.

73. Røttingen J-A et al. *Multi-stakeholder technical meeting on implementation options recommended by the WHO Consultative Expert Working Group on Research & Development (CEWG): Financing and Coordination*. Nonthaburi and Cambridge, MA, International Health Policy Program Thailand and Harvard Global Health Institute, Bellagio, Rockefeller Foundation, 2012.

74. Røttingen J-A et al. Mapping of available health research and development data: what's there, what's missing, and what role is there for a global observatory? *Lancet*, 2013, May 17. pii:S0140-6736(13)61046-6. doi: http://dx.doi.org/10.1016/S0140-6736(13)61046-6

75. Chirac P, Torreele E. Global framework on essential health R&D. *Lancet*, 2006,367:1560-1561. doi: http://dx.doi.org/10.1016/S0140-6736(06)68672-8 PMID:16698397

76. Braine T. Race against time to develop new antibiotics. *Bulletin of the World Health Organization*, 2011,89:88-89. doi: http://dx.doi.org/10.2471/BLT.11.030211 PMID:21346918

77. Leroy JL. et al. Current priorities in health research funding and lack of impact on the number of child deaths per year. *American Journal of Public Health*, 2007,97:219-223. doi: http://dx.doi.org/10.2105/AJPH.2005.083287 PMID:17194855

78. Rothwell PM. Funding for practice-oriented clinical research. *Lancet*, 2006,368:262-266. doi: http://dx.doi.org/10.1016/S0140-6736(06)69010-7 PMID:16860680

79. Zachariah R et al. The 2012 world health report 'no health without research': the endpoint needs to go beyond publication outputs. *Tropical Medicine & International Health*, 2012,17:1409-1411. doi: http://dx.doi.org/10.1111/j.1365-3156.2012.03072.x

80. Brooks A et al. Implementing new health interventions in developing countries: why do we lose a decade or more? *BioMed Central Public Health.*, 2012,12:683. doi: http://dx.doi.org/10.1186/1471-2458-12-683 PMID:22908877

81. Bennett S, Ssengooba F. Closing the gaps: from science to action in maternal, newborn, and child health in Africa. *PLoS Medicine*, 2010,7:e1000298. doi: http://dx.doi.org/10.1371/journal.pmed.1000298 PMID:20613861

82. Nordling L. African nations vow to support science. *Nature*, 2010,465:994-995. doi: http://dx.doi.org/10.1038/465994a PMID:20577179

83. *The Paris Declaration on Aid Effectiveness and the Accra Agenda for Action*. Paris, Organisation for Economic Co-operation and Development, 2013 (http://www.oecd.org/dac/effectiveness/parisdeclarationandaccraagendaforaction.htm, accessed 16 March 2013).

84. *Fourth High Level Forum on Aid Effectiveness*. Busan, Global Partnership for Effective Development Cooperation, 2011. (www.aideffectiveness.org/busanhlf4/, accessed 14 March 2013).

85. Oxman AD et al. A framework for mandatory impact evaluation to ensure well informed public policy decisions. *Lancet*, 2010,375:427-431. doi: http://dx.doi.org/10.1016/S0140-6736(09)61251-4 PMID:20113827

86. *Evaluation for development* (web page). Ottawa, International Development Research Centre, 2012. (http://www.idrc.ca/EN/Programs/Evaluation/Pages/default.aspx, accessed 16 March 2013).

87. Health Economics Research Group, Brunel University. Office of Health Economics, RAND Europe. *Medical research. What's it worth? Estimating the economic benefits from medical research in the UK*. London, UK Evaluation Forum, 2008.

88. *First Funding. Exceptional returns. The economic value of America's investment in medical research*. New York, NY, Albert & Mary Lasker Foundation, 2000.

89. *Exceptional returns: the value of investing in health R&D in Australia II*. Canberra, The Australian Society for Medical Research, 2008.

90. Johnston SC et al. Effect of a US National Institutes of Health programme of clinical trials on public health and costs. *Lancet*, 2006,367:1319-1327. doi: http://dx.doi.org/10.1016/S0140-6736(06)68578-4 PMID:16631910

91. Yazdizadeh B, Majdzadeh R, Salmasian H. Systematic review of methods for evaluating healthcare research economic impact. *Health Research Policy and Systems*, 2010,8:6. doi: http://dx.doi.org/10.1186/1478-4505-8-6 PMID:20196839

92. Donovan C, Hanney S. The 'Payback Framework' explained. *Research Evaluation*, 2011,20:181-183. doi: http://dx.doi.org/10.3152/095820211X13118583635756

93. Wooding S et al. Payback arising from research funding: evaluation of the Arthritis Research Campaign. *Rheumatology*, 2005,44:1145-1156. doi: http://dx.doi.org/10.1093/rheumatology/keh708 PMID:16049052

94. Hanney S et al. An assessment of the impact of the NHS Health Technology Assessment Programme. *Health Technology Assessment*, 2007,11:iii-iv, ix–xi, 1–180. PMID:18031652

95. Oortwijn WJ et al. Assessing the impact of health technology assessment in the Netherlands. *International Journal of Technology Assessment in Health Care*, 2008,24:259-269. doi: http://dx.doi.org/10.1017/S0266462308080355 PMID:18601793

96. Kwan P et al. A systematic evaluation of payback of publicly funded health and health services research in Hong Kong. *BMC Health Services Research*, 2007,7:121. doi: http://dx.doi.org/10.1186/1472-6963-7-121 PMID:17662157

97. Buxton M, Hanney S. How can payback from health services research be assessed? *Journal of Health Services Research & Policy*, 1996,1:35-43. PMID:10180843

98. Nason E et al. *Health research – making an impact. The economic and social benefits of HRB funded research*. Dublin, Health Research Board, 2008.

99. Stevens AJ et al. The role of public-sector research in the discovery of drugs and vaccines. *The New England Journal of Medicine*, 2011,364:535-541. doi: http://dx.doi.org/10.1056/NEJMsa1008268 PMID:21306239

100. Whitworth JA et al. Strengthening capacity for health research in Africa. *Lancet*, 2008,372:1590-1593. doi: http://dx.doi.org/10.1016/S0140-6736(08)61660-8 PMID:18984193

101. Chan M. *Best days for public health are ahead of us, says WHO Director-General. Address to the Sixty-fifth World Health Assembly, Geneva, 21 May 2012*. Geneva, World Health Organization, 2012. (http://www.who.int/dg/speeches/2012/wha_20120521, accessed 14 March 2013).

102. Frenk J, Chen L. Overcoming gaps to advance global health equity: a symposium on new directions for research. *Health Research Policy and Systems*, 2011,9:11. doi: http://dx.doi.org/10.1186/1478-4505-9-11 PMID:21342523

103. Thorsteinsdottir H, ed. *South-South collaboration in health biotechnology: growing partnerships amongst developing countries*. New Delhi and Ottawa, Academic Foundation and International Development Research Centre, 2012.

How research contributes to
universal health coverage

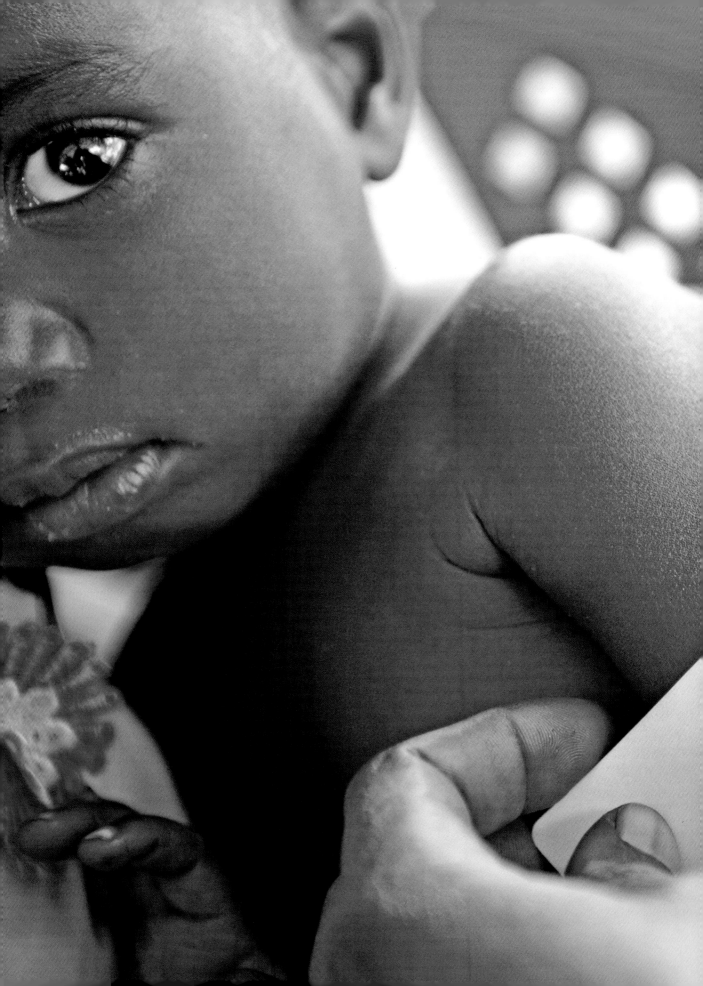

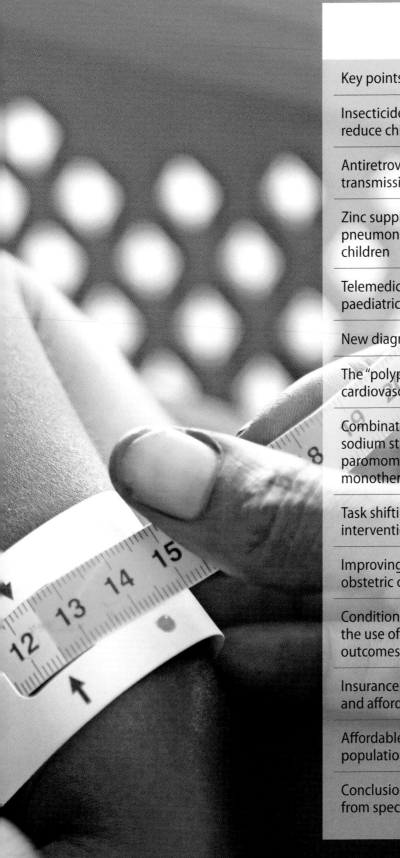

Chapter 3

A health worker measures the mid-upper arm circumference of a child at a nutrition centre in Koubigou, Chad. The yellow on the armband indicates that the child is malnourished (© UNICEF/NYHQ2011-2139/Esteve).

Key points

- Research illuminates the path to universal health coverage and to better health. This chapter illustrates this with 12 case-studies which investigate questions on issues ranging from the prevention and control of specific diseases to the functioning of health systems.

- Several case-studies show how the path to universal health coverage is linked with progress towards the health-related MDGs, which concern maternal and child health and the control of major communicable diseases.

- Research for universal health coverage addresses questions on three levels. First, what is the nature of the health problem, e.g. is it disease-related or health-system related? Second, what specific question is being asked, and where is this question placed in the cycle of research from understanding causes to applying solutions? Third, what is the most appropriate study design for addressing the question at hand?

- The case-studies illustrate the questions on all three levels. In particular, they highlight the range of methods that are commonly used in health research, from observational studies to randomized controlled trials.

- These examples also lead to some general conclusions about research for universal health coverage. They illustrate the diversity of problems for which research can offer solutions, the benefits of having evidence from multiple sources, the nature of the research cycle, the relationship between study design and strength of inference, the challenge of applying research findings from one setting to another, and the link between research, policy and practice.

3

How research contributes to universal health coverage

Chapter 2 showed how research for health in general, and for universal health coverage in particular, has been increasing around the world, albeit unevenly. Turning now to the findings of research, this chapter illustrates, with selected case-studies, how research can address a wide range of questions about universal health coverage and provide answers that can guide health policy and practice.

In selecting and describing the case-studies, we recognize a hierarchy of investigations on three levels. The first level is about identifying the nature of the health problem. The focus might be on a specific disease (such as diabetes, hypertension, tuberculosis or HIV/AIDS), or on the functioning of an element of the health system (such as the health workforce, national laboratory network, or fairness of a health insurance scheme). Covering both diseases and health systems, this chapter focuses on research that helps to make progress, not only towards universal health coverage but also towards achieving the health-related MDGs and sustaining these goals thereafter. The research examples include questions about child health (MDG 4) and maternal health (MDG 5), and about HIV/AIDS, tuberculosis and malaria (MDG 6). The chapter also discusses noncommunicable diseases, the functioning of health systems, and financial barriers to health care.

The second level is about defining the research question, classifying it and placing it within the cycle of research (Box 2.3). The case-studies in this chapter are organized according to the classification proposed by the United Kingdom Clinical Research Collaboration, spanning eight categories from "underpinning research" (i.e. basic or fundamental research) to health policy and systems research (Box 2.2) (1, 2). The 12 case-studies listed in Table 3.1 are ordered according to this scheme. This collection of case-studies falls into categories 3–8 in Box 2.2, because "underpinning research" (category 1) and "disease etiology", (category 2) are less directly relevant to universal health coverage than the other categories.

The studies in this chapter have been selected to reflect a wide variety of situations, approaches and conditions, ranging from the "prevention of diseases and promotion of well-being" to "health policy and systems research". They are placed all around the research cycle described in Chapter 2. The investigations were done mainly in low-and middle-income countries, where the

Table 3.1. The case-studies of research for universal health coverage described in this chapter

Case-study number	Research classification (category in Box 2.2)	Identified health problem	Study type	Country	Main findings	Implications for universal health coverage
1	Prevention of disease and conditions, and promotion of well-being (category 3)	High *malaria* transmission and mortality.	Meta-analysis of household survey data (3)	22 African countries	Use of ITNs was associated with reductions in malaria parasitaemia and mortality in young children.	The evidence supported efforts to scale up and maintain ITN coverage by showing the effect of a proven intervention in a real-life setting (4).
2	Prevention of disease and conditions, and promotion of well-being (category 3)	High rates of sexual transmission of *HIV* infections.	Multicountry randomized controlled trial (5)	Nine countries in Africa, Asia, Latin America and North America	Early ART initiation significantly reduced rates of sexual transmission of HIV.	The study supported the strategic use of ART to reduce the spread of HIV infection and strengthened the evidence base for the development of new global policy and guidelines on use of ART for treatment and prevention of HIV.
3	Prevention of disease and conditions, and promotion of well-being (category 3)	Childhood morbidity and mortality from diarrhoea and respiratory infections is high and may be prevented by *zinc supplementation*.	Randomized controlled trial (6)	Bangladesh	Weekly zinc supplements protected against episodes of pneumonia, diarrhoea and suppurative otitis media, and also prevented deaths.	This evidence added weight to the UNICEF/WHO management recommendations to use zinc supplements for diarrhoea. It also showed the additional benefit of zinc in the management of respiratory diseases.
4	Detection, screening and diagnosis (category 4)	Quality of *paediatric care* is often poor in conflict settings.	Prospective cohort study with historical controls (7)	Somalia	Use of telemedicine technology improved the quality of paediatric care in a hospital setting.	Telemedicine could be used to provide expertise in hard-to-reach and conflict-affected populations that do not have direct access to health services.
5	Detection, screening and diagnosis (category 4)	Common diagnostic tests for *tuberculosis* are insensitive and cannot detect drug resistance.	Validity assessment of a new diagnostic test (8)	Azerbaijan India, Peru, South Africa	Xpert® MTB/RIF, a fully-automated nucleic acid amplification assay, provided higher diagnostic sensitivity for pulmonary TB and rapid detection of rifampicin resistance.	WHO recommended the use of the Xpert® MTB/RIF assay in 2010. By September 2012, 898 Xpertinstruments had been procured in the public sector in 73 of the 145 countries eligible for concessional pricing.

continues …

... continued

Case-study number	Research classification (category in Box 2.2)	Identified health problem	Study type	Country	Main findings	Implications for universal health coverage
6	Development of treatments and therapeutic interventions (category 5)	Cardiovascular disease is a major *noncommunicable disease* and a global public health problem.	Randomized controlled trial (9)	India	"Polypill" – a single pill containing a combination of drugs – effectively reduced multiple risk factors for cardiovascular disease.	Use of the polypill may reduce cardiovascular morbidity and death when integrated with other preventive activities such as exercise and healthy diets.
7	Evaluation of treatments and therapeutic interventions (category 6)	*Visceral leishmaniasis* is the second largest parasitic killer in the world after malaria, but treatment options are limited.	Multicountry randomized controlled trial (10)	Ethiopia, Kenya, Sudan, Uganda	Combination treatment with SSG and PM was effective, was of shorter duration and was associated with reduced risk of development of drug resistance.	The evidence led to a WHO recommendation that SSG and PM could be used as a first-line combination treatment for visceral leishmaniasis in East Africa.
8	Management of diseases and conditions (category 7)	Lack of *qualified health staff affects* coverage of child survival interventions.	Multicountry observational study (11)	Bangladesh, Brazil, Uganda, United Republic of Tanzania	Task shifting from health workers with longer duration of training to those with shorter duration of training did not compromise quality of care for IMCI.	Task shifting is an effective strategy for strengthening health systems, and for increasing coverage of IMCI and other child survival interventions, in underserved and resource-limited areas faced with staff shortages.
9	Health policy and systems research (category 8)	High *maternal mortality* in Africa.	Retrospective cohort study (12)	Burundi	Provision of access to emergency obstetric care was associated with a rapid and substantial reduction in maternal mortality in a rural district.	Emergency obstetric care is one way, among others, to achieve MDG 5 in rural Africa.
10	Health policy and systems research (category 8)	*Financial barriers* negatively influence access to and utilization of health services.	Systematic review (13)	Brazil, Colombia, Honduras, Malawi, Mexico, Nicaragua	CCTs increased health service utilization and were associated with improved health outcomes.	CCT schemes are a financial incentive to increase demand for and utilization of health services by reducing or eliminating financial barriers to access.
11	Health policy and systems research (category 8)	*Out-of-pocket expenses* and catastrophic household expenditures are barriers to achieving universal health coverage.	Cluster randomized trial (14)	Mexico	A public national health insurance scheme reduced out-of-pocket expenses and catastrophic expenditures, with benefits reaching poorer households.	This national health insurance scheme led to Mexico celebrating the achievement of universal health coverage in 2011.

continues ...

... *continued*

Case-study number	Research classification (category in Box 2.2)	Identified health problem	Study type	Country	Main findings	Implications for universal health coverage
12	Health policy and systems research (category 8)	Potentially *unsustainable financing* of health systems in countries with ageing populations.	Quantitative forecasts of public health expenditure associated with ageing, 2010–2060 (1)	Czech Republic, Germany, Hungary, Netherlands, Slovenia	Projected increases in public health expenditure due to ageing are moderate and are falling from the 2030s onwards.	Although ageing is not expected to incur large extra costs, systems of health care, long-term care and welfare in European countries must adapt to population ageing.

ART, antiretroviral therapy; CCT, conditional cash transfer; HIV, human immunodeficiency virus; IMCI, integrated management of childhood illness; ITN, insecticide-treated bed net; MDG, Millennium Development Goal; MDG 5, Millennium Development Goal 5 – reduce maternal mortality by 75% between 1990 and 2015; PM, paromomycin sulfate; SSG, sodium stibogluconate; TB, tuberculosis; UNICEF, United Nations Children's Fund; WHO, World Health Organization.

gap between the present coverage of health services and universal health coverage is greatest. In keeping with the realities of doing research, the evidence is of varying quality and has variably influenced the development or adjustment of health policies.

For each type of question, the investigation begins with understanding the problem, proceeds with the development of a solution, and then evaluates the feasibility, cost, effectiveness and cost–effectiveness of that solution. Evaluation leads to further questions, and so another cycle of research or evaluation begins (Box 2.3). As the evidence improves through repeated cycles of research, changes to policy advice can be expected too.

The third level is about designing the investigation. The task is to select the most appropriate methods for collecting reliable information in the most rigorous way, producing evidence that will answer the research questions at hand and ultimately improve health coverage, either through the implementation of new interventions or by developing new policies. Study designs range from observational investigations that can have important qualitative components (e.g. among targeted groups of patients or health-care workers) to comparisons of interventions in which the primary outcomes are determined by quantitative methods (Table 3.2) (15). Some complex designs mix qualitative and quantitative elements (16). The choice of design influences the feasibility, cost and duration of the study as well as the potential reliability (validity) and usefulness. Observational studies are sometimes quicker, cheaper and easier to conduct than formal experiments but may be less conclusive because they are especially prone to bias and may ultimately be misleading (Box 2.3), so there is a compromise in study design. The choice of methods may depend on the likelihood and importance of obtaining results that could eventually influence health policy.

Emerging from the 12 examples that follow are some general features of research for universal health coverage. These are identified at the end of the chapter.

Table 3.2.   Overview of research study designs

Study type[a,b]	Studying	Method to organize the study	How conclusions are derived
Systematic reviews of experiments[c]	Primary studies	Systematic search	Summarize strength of evidence
Experiments using random allocation (RCTs) or minimization[d,e]	Enrollees	Assign to study group using randomization or minimization	Intervene, measure, follow and compare
Experiments using other allocation methods	Enrollees	Assign to study group through other methods	Intervene, measure, follow and compare
Systematic reviews of observations w/ or w/o experiments	Primary studies	Systematic search	Summarize strength of evidence
Cohort study (prospective or historical retrospective)	Enrollees or population[f]	Group by presence or absence of characteristic such as risk factor	Follow and compare
Case-control (retrospective)	Population	Group by outcome of interest	Compare characterstics (e.g. exposure)
Cross-sectional[g]	Population	Group assessed at a single point in time	Assess prevalence of characteristic and association with an outcome
Case series	Patients	Observe and report	Describe treatment and outcome
Case report	Individual patient	Observe and report	Describe treatment and outcome

RCTs, randomized controlled trials.

[a]   The choice of study type frequently depends upon the health care question.

[b]   All studies should be critically appraised for validity (bias and chance) and evaluated for usefulness.

[c]   Non-systematic reviews and other observations not included in this table .

[d]   In general, valid experiments (e.g. RCTs) are the most reliable designs for investigating cause and effect in medical and public health interventions.

[e]   "Minimization" is a method of adaptive allocation that aims to minimize imbalances between prognostic variables of patients assigned to different treatment groups.

[f]   A "population" is typically a subset of a larger population.

[g]   Some of these general study types have different names (e.g. a cross-sectional study may also be called a prevalence study).

Reproduced, by permission of the publisher, from Stuart ME, Strite SA, Delfini Group LLC (www.delfini.org).

Case-study 1

Insecticide-treated mosquito nets to reduce childhood mortality: a systematic analysis of survey data from 22 sub-Saharan African countries

The need for research

By killing or repelling mosquitoes, insecticide-treated bed nets (ITNs, Fig. 3.1) protect the individuals sleeping under them from malaria. By killing mosquitoes, they should also reduce malaria transmission in the community (4).

Randomized controlled trials conducted in sub-Saharan Africa in a range of malaria-endemic settings have provided robust evidence of the efficacy of ITNs in reducing malaria parasite prevalence and incidence and all-cause child mortality (17, 18). Such trials showed that ITNs can reduce *Plasmodium falciparum* prevalence among children younger than five years of age by 13% and malaria deaths by 18%. As a result,

Fig. 3.1.   Household use of insecticide-treated mosquito bed nets

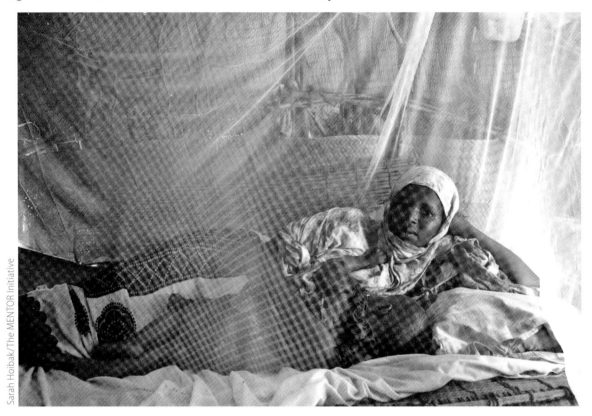

Sarah Hoibak/The MENTOR Initiative

widespread provision of ITNs became central to global efforts to control malaria. In 2005, the World Health Assembly set a target of providing ITNs to at least 80% of persons at risk of malaria by 2010. Progress towards this goal has varied among countries, although several countries in sub-Saharan Africa scaled up the proportion of households that own ITNs from almost zero to more than 60% with support from international donors (*19*). There was a dramatic increase in funding for malaria control from US$ 100 million in 2003 to US$ 1.5 billion in 2010, most of which was invested in sub-Saharan Africa (*4*). Between 2004 and 2010, more than 400 million bed nets were delivered (290 million since 2008) – sufficient to cover almost 80% of populations at risk of malaria in Africa (*20*).

In contrast with the findings of controlled trials, ITNs may be less effective in routine use because the insecticidal effect wears off, or nets may be used inappropriately or become damaged. The impact of ITNs, as used routinely, on malaria and childhood mortality is therefore uncertain.

Study design

A meta-analysis of six Malaria Indicator Surveys and one Demographic and Health Survey was carried out to determine the association between household ITN ownership and the prevalence of malaria parasitaemia. The reduction in child mortality was further assessed using data from 29 Demographic and Health Surveys undertaken in 22 countries of sub-Saharan Africa (*3*).

Summary of findings

Investigators pooled the results of the individual surveys and found a 20% (95% confidence interval, CI: 3–35%) reduction in prevalence of malaria parasitaemia associated with household ownership of at least one ITN, as compared with no ITN. Sleeping under an ITN the previous night was associated with a 24% (95% CI: 1–42%) reduction in the prevalence of malaria parasitaemia. Ownership of at least one ITN was associated with a reduction in mortality in children under five years of age of 23% (95% CI: 13–31%), which was consistent with that seen in the randomized controlled trials.

The accuracy of these findings may be affected by the observational study design. For instance, it is possible that people who owned ITNs shared other characteristics that contributed to the reduction in parasitaemia prevalence and childhood deaths. Possible confounding factors include the use of anti-malarial drugs, better use and recourse to health care, and household wealth.

Towards universal health coverage

Despite the caveats, these findings suggest that the beneficial effects of ITNs demonstrated in clinical trials are also obtained in routine use. As resources for global health become more limited, this evidence should reassure donors and national programmes that the investments made so far have been effective in controlling malaria. The efficacy of ITNs is substantially reduced after 2–3 years due to net damage and the loss of insecticidal effects, and there is therefore a need to find ways of replacing or re-impregnating nets (*21*). The evidence from this study justifies continued efforts to scale up ITN coverage in sub-Saharan Africa and highlights the importance of maintaining ITN coverage in countries where they have already been distributed widely.

Main conclusions

- Under routine use in African households, the effectiveness of ITNs in reducing malaria parasitaemia and child mortality

was consistent with that seen in clinical trials.

- This evidence supports continued efforts to expand and then maintain the coverage of ITNs.

Case-study 2

Antiretroviral therapy to prevent sexual transmission of HIV: a randomized controlled trial of serodiscordant couples in nine countries

The need for research

By the end of 2011, more than eight million people in low- and middle-income countries were estimated to be receiving antiretroviral therapy (ART). On the basis of current ART eligibility criteria (all HIV-infected people with ≤ 350 CD4 cells/uL), these numbers represent a global coverage of 56% compared with 6% in 2003 (*22*).

Despite this achievement, HIV/AIDS continues to impose a major burden on health: an estimated 2.5 million people were newly infected with HIV in 2011 and 1.7 million people died from AIDS (*22*). It is clear that the HIV/AIDS epidemic will not be brought under control without markedly reducing HIV transmission and the incidence of new infections.

Study design

In nine countries in Africa, Asia, Latin America and North America, 1763 couples were enrolled in a randomized placebo-controlled trial (HPTN 052) in which one partner was HIV-positive and the other was HIV-negative (i.e. serodiscordant couples) (*5*). HIV-infected persons whose CD4-lymphocyte counts were between 350 and 550 cells/uL were assigned to receive ART immediately (early ART group) or after the CD4 count had declined to ≤ 250 cells/uL or after the development of an AIDS-related illness (delayed ART group). HIV-uninfected partners were encouraged to return for all visits to receive counselling on risk reduction and the use of condoms, for treatment of sexually transmitted infections, and for management of other medical conditions. The primary prevention end point was HIV transmission in HIV-negative partners.

Summary of findings

A total of 39 HIV transmissions were observed (incidence rate 1.2 per 100 person-years; 95% CI: 0.9–1.7), of which 28 were virologically linked to the infected partner (incidence rate 0.9 per 100 person-years; 95% CI: 0.6–1.3). Of the 28 linked HIV transmissions, only one occurred in the early ART group and 27 occurred in the late ART group, giving a 96% (95% CI: 72–99%) reduction in the risk of HIV transmission (hazard ratio 0.04; 95% CI: 0.01–0.27, Fig. 3.2). Early ART was also associated with a reduction in individual HIV-related clinical events, mainly those due to extra-pulmonary tuberculosis (hazard ratio 0.59; 95% CI: 0.40–0.88).

Previous observational cohort studies had suggested that early start of ART had an HIV-prevention effect but this was the first randomized controlled trial to establish definitive proof. The most likely mechanism is sustained suppression of HIV in genital secretions. The study provides strong support for the early use of ART in serodiscordant couples as one component of a comprehensive public health strategy to reduce the spread of HIV that includes behaviour change, use of condoms, male circumcision, female ART-based microbicides and pre-exposure ART prophylaxis.

Towards universal health coverage

The HPTN 052 study was voted "breakthrough of the year" in 2011 by the journal *Science*, galvanizing efforts to end the global HIV/AIDS epidemic (*23*). In April 2012, WHO issued guidance on HIV testing and counselling for couples, recommending that HIV serodiscordant couples with CD4 counts ≥ 350 cells/uL should be offered

Fig. 3.2. **HIV transmission linked to partners within serodiscordant couples, with respect to the year since entering the trial, and according to whether ART was given early or with a delay (inset)**

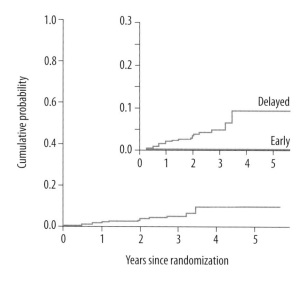

ART, antiretroviral therapy; HIV, human immunodeficiency virus.
Adapted, by permission of the publisher, from Cohen et al. (*5*).

ART to reduce HIV transmission to uninfected partners (*24*). WHO also published a programmatic update on the use of ART for treating pregnant women and preventing HIV infection in infants, including the use of so-called Option B+. This option provides ART to HIV-infected women, regardless of CD4 count, as a simple strategy to eliminate HIV infection in infants while at the same time protecting the health of the mother, father and subsequent children. Malawi was the first country to propose such an approach, and provided Option B+ to over 35 000 HIV-infected pregnant women in the first 12 months of implementation (*25*). HPTN 052 now provides additional, strong scientific justification for this intervention. In mid-2012 WHO released a discussion paper on the strategic use of antiretroviral drugs to help end the HIV epidemic, providing the rationale for developing new consolidated global ART guidelines in 2013 which will emphasize the efficacy of ART for both treatment and prevention of HIV (26).

A series of questions remain to be answered before this intervention can be taken to scale. Among them are whether HIV-infected people who are asymptomatic will be willing to take ART for prevention, whether this approach will increase the risk of drug resistance, and how health services will cope with the added costs and burden of health care.

Main conclusions

- The provision of ART early in the course of HIV infection reduces sexual transmission of the virus between members of serodiscordant couples.
- Early ART can be used as part of a public health strategy to reduce the incidence and spread of HIV infection.
- These research findings have indirectly strengthened the evidence for other complementary approaches to the prevention of HIV infection, including prevention of vertical transmission of HIV from mothers to children.

Case-study 3

Zinc supplements to reduce pneumonia and diarrhoea in young children: a randomized controlled trial in an urban, low-income population in Bangladesh

The need for research
Zinc is a vital micronutrient in humans for protein synthesis and cell growth. Zinc deficiency is highly prevalent in low- and middle-income countries and affected populations are at an increased risk of growth retardation, diarrhoeal diseases, respiratory tract infections and

malaria. Zinc deficiency may be associated with around 800 000 excess global deaths annually among children under five years of age, including deaths attributable to diarrhoea (176 000), pneumonia (406 000) and malaria (176 000) (27). Micronutrient supplements (such as zinc) are therefore potentially important interventions in the context of reaching MDGs 4, 5 and 6.

Several hospital- and community-based randomized trials have shown the beneficial effects of zinc supplementation in reducing the number of episodes of diarrhoea and pneumonia as well as reducing the severity of illness (28, 29). Given the benefits of zinc supplementation, the United Nations Children's Fund (UNICEF) and WHO issued a statement in 2004 that all children with diarrhoea in developing countries should be treated with zinc (30).

However, several questions remain. Research on zinc supplements for the prevention of diarrhoea and pneumonia had mostly included children older than two years of age, while younger children might in fact be more vulnerable to such morbidity. What, therefore, would the effect of zinc supplementation be in younger children? In most of the previous studies, zinc was given on a daily basis, and this might be far less acceptable or feasible than a once-weekly dose. In addition, long-term intake of zinc could adversely affect iron and copper metabolism, both of which are also essential micronutrients. It was felt that answers to these questions would help guide international policy on the use of zinc.

Study design
A randomized controlled trial was conducted among a poor urban population in Dhaka, Bangladesh, to determine if a large weekly dose of zinc (70 mg) would reduce the frequency of clinical pneumonia, diarrhoea, and other morbidity in children younger than two years of age (6). The effects of zinc on growth, haemoglobin concentrations and serum copper were also measured. Children aged from 60 days to 12 months were randomly assigned zinc or placebo orally once

Table 3.3. **Number of diagnoses made in clinics by medical officers in the zinc and placebo groups, Dhaka, Bangladesh**

	Zinc (child-years = 427)[a]	Placebo (child-years = 511)[a]	Relative risk (95% confidence interval)	P-value
Diarrhoea	1881	2407	0.94 (0.88–0.99)	0.030
Upper respiratory infection	4834	6294	0.92 (0.88–0.97)	0.001
Reactive airways disease or bronchiolitis	232	314	0.88 (0.79–0.99)	0.042
Suppurative otitis media	394	572	0.58 (0.41–0.82)	0.002
Pneumonia	199	286	0.83 (0.73–0.95)	0.004
Severe pneumonia	18	42	0.51 (0.30–0.88)	0.016
Death	2	14	0.15 (0.03–0.67)	0.013

[a] Indicates child-years of follow-up.
Reproduced, by permission of the publisher, from Brooks et al. (6).

weekly for 12 months. Children were assessed weekly by research staff for the primary outcomes of pneumonia and diarrhoea using a standardized procedure. Secondary outcomes included rates of other respiratory tract infections.

Summary of findings

A total of 809 children were assigned zinc and 812 assigned placebo. There were significantly fewer incidents of pneumonia in the zinc group compared with the placebo group (199 versus 286; relative risk, RR: 0.83; 95% CI: 0.73–0.95). A significant but modest decrease was observed in the incidence of diarrhoea (1881 cases versus 2407; RR: 0.94; 95% CI: 0.88–0.99). All other illnesses (otitis media, reactive airways disease and bronchiolitis) were significantly less frequent in the zinc group compared with the placebo group (Table 3.3). There were two deaths in the zinc group and 14 in the placebo group. There were no pneumonia-related deaths in the zinc group, but 10 occurred in the placebo group. The zinc group had a small gain in height at 10 months. Serum copper and haemoglobin concentrations were not adversely affected after 10 months of zinc supplementation.

Towards universal health coverage

These findings showed that zinc supplements among young children had a substantial protective effect against episodes of pneumonia and suppurative otitis media and, most importantly, an 85% reduction in mortality owing to prevention of pneumonia-related deaths.

These findings have provided evidence for extending the 2004 UNICEF/WHO management recommendations for the use of zinc for respiratory disease control (30). There have been several other policy implications. Otitis media is a common paediatric infection in resource-limited settings and has important clinical sequelae. By reducing the incidence of otitis media, zinc could reduce hearing-related disability and treatment costs and thus improve the quality of life.

Weekly dosing in young children is also an important step forward in reducing pill counts and enhancing the practical aspects of programmatic management of zinc supplementation. Further studies are now required to assess the optimum dose and length of protection after weekly zinc supplementation.

Main conclusions

- Zinc supplementation among children under two years of age has a substantial protective effect against pneumonia, suppurative otitis media and pneumonia-related mortality. Treatment with zinc also has an effect (albeit modest) on reducing the frequency of diarrhoea and improving growth.

- Once-weekly dosing of zinc was found to be feasible and safe. It was associated with potential programmatic advantages and no measurable negative impact on serum level of copper and haemoglobin.

Case-study 4

Telemedicine to improve the quality of paediatric care: an operational research study in Somalia

The need for research

Somalia has been ravaged by war for over two decades, and health facilities in the country are suffering from a serious shortage of specialist doctors. Health care is provided by a limited number of Somali clinicians who, through the circumstances of war, have had little or no opportunity to pursue continuing education, have virtually no on-site supervision by senior clinicians, and lack access to medical supplies and equipment. The quality of care, particularly for ill children admitted to hospital wards, is a major concern. Achieving universal health coverage means reaching remote locations and conflict-affected populations where the challenges of dilapidated infrastructure and the shortage of qualified, skilled human resources are enormous.

One solution to bridging the gap in expertise in such settings is to use information and communications technology in the form of telemedicine (*31–34*). Telemedicine means "medicine at a distance" and the rationale for introducing this in Somalia is simple – export the expertise (though not the experts) to Somalia (*33*).

Study design

A prospective observational cohort study assessed the impact of the introduction of telemedicine on the quality of paediatric care. The added value, as perceived by local clinicians using the service, was also assessed using a questionnaire (*7*). The study site was the paediatric ward of a district hospital (Guri'el hospital) serving a population of about 327 000 inhabitants. This hospital housed the only paediatric inpatient facility within a radius of 250 km. The telemedicine involved a "real-time" audiovisual exchange of information on paediatric cases between clinicians in Somalia and a specialist paediatrician located in Nairobi, Kenya. The equipment included a mobile camera, a microphone device and a loudspeaker linked to a computer in the paediatric ward in Somalia and a similar configuration in a consultation room in Kenya. The two sites were connected through a broadband Internet service (Fig. 3.3). Impact on quality of care was assessed by comparing the initial diagnosis and prescription (initial management) of each paediatric case with the final diagnosis and treatment (final management) made by the specialist paediatrician, and by comparing adverse hospital outcomes for a period with telemedicine (the intervention year, 2011) with outcomes for a period without telemedicine (the control year, 2010). A questionnaire was also used to gather the perceptions of clinicians on the added value of telemedicine.

Fig. 3.3. **Consultation room and specialist paediatrician in Nairobi, Kenya, conducting a telemedicine consultation with colleagues in Guri'el hospital, Somalia**

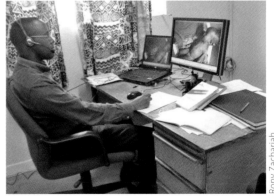

Rony Zachariah

Summary of findings

Of 3920 paediatric admissions, 346 (9%) were referred to the telemedicine service. In 222 children (64% of those referred), a significant change was made to initial case management by the specialist paediatrician, and in 88 children (25% of those referred) a life-threatening condition that had initially been missed was diagnosed. Telemedicine in these cases served as a life-saving intervention (Table 3.4). Over a one-year period there was a progressive improvement in the capacity of clinicians to manage complicated cases, as demonstrated by a significant linear decrease in changes to initial case management for meningitis and convulsions (92% to 29%, $P = 0.001$), lower respiratory tract infections (75% to 45%, $P = 0.02$) and complicated malnutrition (86% to 40%, $P = 0.002$) (Fig. 3.4). Loss

of interest among those using telemedicine is unlikely to explain this finding as all children with the described conditions were systematically referred for telemedicine according to the study protocol and cases were reviewed by the same specialist physician. Adverse outcomes (deaths and losses to follow-up) on paediatric wards decreased by 30% between 2010 (without telemedicine) and 2011 (with telemedicine) (odds ratio 0.70; 95% CI: 0.57– 0.88). All seven clinicians involved with telemedicine rated it as having high added value in improving the recognition of risk signs and prescription practices.

Table 3.4. **Life-threatening conditions that were initially missed and that telemedicine helped to diagnose, Guri'el hospital paediatric ward, Somalia, January–December 2011**

Life-threatening conditions diagnosed through telemedicine	No (%)
Bacterial meningitis and tuberculous meningitis	39 (44)
Pulmonary tuberculosis with severe pleural and/or pericardial effusions	11 (13)
Neonatal septicaemia	11 (13)
Septicaemia/septic shock	6 (7)
Congestive cardiac failure	5 (6)
Severe perinatal asphyxia	3 (3)
Necrotizing enterocolitis	2 (2)
Severe septic arthritis	2 (2)
Severe pyelonephritis	2 (2)
Others	7 (8)
TOTAL	**88 (100%)**

Reproduced, by permission of the publisher, from Zachariah et al. (*7*).

Fig. 3.4. **Decreasing trends in changes to initial case management made after telemedicine consultations with a specialist in Kenya (expressed as a percentage of all cases), Guri'l hospital, Somalia, January–December 2011**

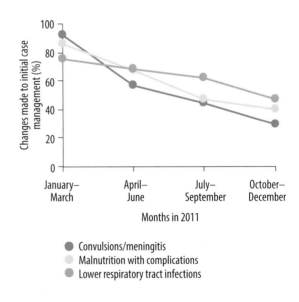

Adapted, by permission of the publisher, from Zachariah et al. (*7*).

Towards universal health coverage

Although this is an observational rather than an experimental study, the findings suggest that telemedicine can provide clinical expertise to remote and inaccessible areas. However, the effectiveness, feasibility and acceptability of introducing such technology, and its impact on improving access to and quality of care, in similar and post-conflict settings need to be evaluated, ideally with a more rigorous experimental approach (*35*).

Main conclusions

- Efforts towards achieving universal health coverage must include people who are hard to reach and those who are affected by conflict.
- In Somalia, telemedicine technology reduced adverse paediatric ward outcomes (deaths and losses to follow-up) by 30% between 2010 (without telemedicine) and 2011 (with telemedicine).
- Telemedicine is a way to bring medical expertise to remote health services without relocating the experts themselves.

Case-study 5

New diagnostics for tuberculosis: a validity assessment of the Xpert® MTB/RIF assay in Azerbaijan, India, Peru and South Africa

The need for research

Despite widespread implementation of the WHO Stop TB Strategy, TB remains a major public health problem. In 2011, there were an estimated 8.7 million new TB cases worldwide, of which only 5.8 million (67%) were notified. This is a measure of the gap in service coverage. In the same year, there were an estimated 310 000 cases of multidrug-resistant TB (MDR-TB), resistant to at least isoniazid and rifampicin, among notified

TB patients with pulmonary TB, of which only 60 000 cases were diagnosed and put on treatment (*36*).

A major reason for poor TB case detection and enrolment to treatment is the inadequacy of diagnostic tools. For decades, the mainstay of TB diagnosis has been sputum-smear microscopy for patients with suspected pulmonary TB, followed by chest radiography in those with negative sputum smears. This process is time-consuming, costly for the patient who needs to make multiple journeys to the clinic, and diagnostically insensitive. This is especially true for HIV-infected TB patients, among whom a significant proportion has negative sputum smears and a normal chest X-ray (particularly those with advanced HIV/AIDS disease). Furthermore, smear microscopy cannot diagnose MDR-TB.

Study design

The most revolutionary diagnostic development to date for tuberculosis is a sensitive and specific nucleic acid amplification test, the Xpert® MTB/RIF assay (Cepheid Inc., Sunnyvale, CA, USA), which uses a common platform to diagnose mycobacterium tuberculosis (MTB) and rifampicin resistance (RIF) (Fig. 3.5). The cartridge-based system requires minimal laboratory expertise and fully automated results are available in less than two hours. The performance of Xpert MTB/RIF was assessed in health facilities in Azerbaijan, India, Peru and South Africa (*8*).

Summary of findings

There were 1730 patients with suspected drug-sensitive or multidrug resistant pulmonary tuberculosis, each of whom submitted three sputum specimens, and 1462 eligible patients were included in the main analysis. Using sputum culture as the reference test, the Xpert MTB/RIF assay was specific in 604 of 609 patients without TB (99.2% of negatives detected). The overall sensitivity (% of true positives detected) for one sputum specimen in patients with smear-positive tuberculosis was 97.6% (95% CI: 96.2–98.5). For patients with smear-negative culture-positive

Fig. 3.5.   Xpert® MTB/RIF machine being used in a health facility in South Africa

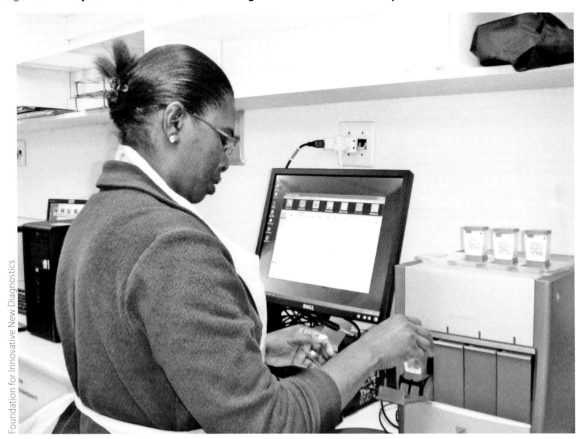

Foundation for Innovative New Diagnostics

TB, sensitivity increased with the number of smears tested (Fig. 3.6). The overall sensitivity and specificity (% of true negatives) for detecting rifampicin resistance was 97.6% (95% CI: 94.4–99.0) and 98.1% (95% CI: 96.5–98.9) respectively.

Towards universal health coverage

On the basis of these and subsequent results, WHO recommended in December 2010 that Xpert MTB/RIF should be used as the initial diagnostic test in persons suspected of having HIV-associated TB and in those at risk of MDR-TB (37). It may also be used as a follow-on test to microscopy, especially for patients with smear-negative specimens (38). As of September 2012, a total of 898 GeneXpert instruments and 1 482 550 Xpert MTB/RIF cartridges had been

procured in the public sector in 73 of the 145 countries eligible for concessional pricing (39). Operational feasibility, accuracy and effectiveness were assessed and were confirmed at district and subdistrict health facilities in Africa, Asia, Europe and South America (40). However, further assessment at more peripheral facilities is required because the machine's performance in these settings depends on operational factors such as cost, temperature, cartridge shelf-life, power supply, maintenance and calibration needs. The public health impact of Xpert MTB/RIF also depends on the link between diagnosis and subsequent treatment.

National TB control programmes need to find optimal diagnostic algorithms tailored to local epidemiological conditions to make the

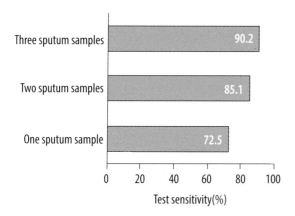

Fig. 3.6.   **Sensitivity of Xpert MTB/RIF assay with multiple smears for smear-negative, culture-positive tuberculosis (commonly seen in HIV-positive individuals)**

HIV, human immunodeficiency virus.
Source: Boehme et al. (8)

best use of Xpert MTB/RIF. This technology and related research have the potential to bring diagnosis closer to patients. Further operational studies are under way to investigate the cost, optimal location and use of the assay within health systems and in combination with other diagnostic tools (41). As investigations of the performance of Xpert MTB/RIF have proliferated, study design also appears to have improved (K Weyer, WHO, personal communication), indicating an instance of technological development boosting the quality of research (38).

Main conclusions

- The Xpert MTB/RIF assay is useful for rapid detection of TB and rifampicin resistance, which is indicative of MDR-TB. The test is particularly useful for detecting TB in patients with HIV infection, thereby allowing the diagnosis of patients earlier in the course of their disease.

- Following WHO recommendations in December 2010, approximately 900 Xpert MTB/RIF instruments had been procured for the public sector in 73 countries by the end of September 2012.

- Further research is under way to confront operational and logistic challenges in laboratory and field areas, and to assess affordability, epidemiological impact and cost–effectiveness.

Case-study 6

The "polypill" to reduce deaths from cardiovascular disease: a randomized controlled trial in India

The need for research

There is a growing global epidemic of noncommunicable diseases – primarily cardiovascular diseases, diabetes, cancer and chronic respiratory diseases. These are responsible for two thirds of the 57 million deaths worldwide each year, with 80% of deaths occurring in low- and middle-income countries. Deaths from noncommunicable diseases are projected to rise from 36 million in 2008 to 52 million in 2030 (42). In response to this epidemic, WHO Member States have agreed on a set of targets to reduce deaths caused by the four main noncommunicable diseases by 25% in people aged 30–70 years by 2025 (43). WHO has proposed 10 targets to reach this goal. One of these targets is drug therapy to reduce the prevalence of risk factors for heart attack and stroke (42).

A combination pill for the prevention of cardiovascular disease was first described in 2000, and shortly afterwards the "polypill" was presented as a strategy to reduce cardiovascular disease (44). The concept is simple. Several different drugs (aspirin, beta blockers, angiotensin-converting-enzyme inhibitors and statins) are available generically and inexpensively to treat several risk factors for cardiovascular disease, particularly ischaemic heart disease. Combining several drugs into a single polypill is appealing because of its simplicity and acceptability, and because one pill is more likely to be taken routinely than several will be.

Methods

In 2009, a phase II double-blind randomized trial was conducted on the effect of a polypill on risk factors in middle-aged persons without cardiovascular disease at 50 centres in India. The study was designated "The Indian Polycap Study" (TIPS) (9). The polypill consisted of a combination of low doses of a thiazide diuretic, atenolol, ramipril, simvastatin and aspirin, and this was compared with single agents or combinations of single agents. The effect of the medication was measured on risk factors, including high blood pressure, elevated cholesterol concentrations and elevated heart rate. Polypill intake was also assessed for feasibility and tolerability.

Summary of findings

A total of 2053 individuals aged 45–80 years without cardiovascular disease and with at least one risk factor were included in the study. The Indian Polycap study reduced systolic blood pressure by 7.4 mmHg (95% CI: 6.1–8.1), diastolic blood pressure by 5.6 mm Hg (95% CI: 4.7–6.4), and low-density lipoprotein cholesterol by 0.70 mmol/L (95% CI: 0.62–0.78). The reduction in heart rate was 7.0 beats per minute on average. These reductions were better or similar to those of single drugs or combinations of single drugs and tolerability was similar to that of other treatments. Effects of the polypill at the wider population level might be affected by adherence. Importantly, a third of the participants in the TIPS study had diabetes mellitus, a population in which the clustering of risk factors is known to be common. Comorbidity offers the potential for targeted treatment, if and when a polypill is used for primary prevention.

Towards universal health coverage

The results of the study showed that each of the components of the polypill reduced the risk of cardiovascular disease. Several other trials have since been carried out to demonstrate the effects of different polypills in reducing blood pressure and cholesterol with generally good results, although issues of adherence and lower-than-expected benefits were encountered (45).

The current evidence needs to be extended by carrying out large phase III trials to investigate the efficacy of the polypill in reducing the incidence of cardiovascular disease and stroke, and mortality associated with these conditions, in large groups of human subjects over much longer periods of time (46). Operational questions pose a challenge to the translation of existing evidence into policy. These questions need to be answered by clinical and observational studies which include: (i) the safety profile and what to do if one component of the polypill is contraindicated or causes a side-effect; (ii) the doses of the various components; and (iii) whether a pill that might be perceived as a magic solution to noncommunicable diseases would lead people to abandon other preventive measures such as appropriate diets, behaviour change and exercise. Research is needed to measure both the potential of such an intervention to reduce the global burden of cardiovascular disease and the intervention's public health merit before policy is developed on the basis of the TIPS study.

Main conclusions

- Early research shows that the Polycap formulation, a single pill that combines several drugs, might be a simple and practical way to reduce multiple risk factors and cardiovascular disease, a major global public health problem.
- There is a need for phase III clinical trials to evaluate more precisely the efficacy of the polypill, and for operational research to assess the feasibility of using this treatment in practice.

- The effect of the polypill needs to be assessed in conjunction with other means of reducing the risk of cardiovascular disease, such as dietary changes, the prevention of tobacco smoking, and physical exercise regimes.

Case-study 7

Combination treatment with sodium stibogluconate (SSG) and paromomycin compared to SSG monotherapy for visceral leishmaniasis: a randomized controlled trial in Ethiopia, Kenya, Sudan and Uganda

The need for research

Human visceral leishmaniasis (VL), also known as *kala-azar*, is a life-threatening parasitic disease caused by *Leishmania donovani* and transmitted by phlebotomine sandflies (Fig. 3.7). VL is the second largest parasitic killer in the world after malaria, with an annual worldwide incidence of approximately 500 000 cases (47). VL is an important disease in Asia (Bangladesh, India, Nepal) and East Africa. In East Africa, the incidence rate is 30 000 cases with 4000 deaths per year (48). The *Leishmania* parasite migrates to internal organs such as the liver, spleen and bone marrow (hence the term "visceral") and, if untreated, will frequently lead to death. Effective measures to eradicate the sandfly are lacking, death rates are high, and there are few affordable and effective treatment options. This situation, along with the fact that there is limited research and drug development for VL, means that VL can be called a "neglected disease".

Treatment for VL in East Africa is primarily limited to the antimonial sodium stibogluconate (SSG), which is efficacious but requires four weeks of hospitalization and daily intramuscular injections and is associated with serious adverse events such as cardiotoxicity. The drug is thus difficult to administer and constitutes a burden both for the patient and for the health system. The parasite is also becoming increasingly resistant to the drug.

The efficacy of an alternative drug, paromomycin sulfate (PM), has been demonstrated in India (49). There is, however, limited information on the efficacy of PM for VL in the African setting where response to treatment may be different. A large observational study of 4263 VL patients in South Sudan showed that a combination of SSG and PM for a shorter period of time (17 days) yielded better results than SSG alone (50). For registration of PM and evaluation of the efficacy of combination treatment with SSG and PM in East Africa, efficacy and safety data were required from a phase III randomized controlled trial.

Study design

A multicentre randomized controlled trial was conducted in four East African countries (Ethiopia, Kenya, Sudan and Uganda) (10). The trial had three arms: (i) SSG monotherapy (a dose of 20 mg/kg/day for 30 days) used as the reference arm; (ii) PM monotherapy (20 mg/kg/day for 21 days); and (iii) a combination of SSG and PM given for a shorter period (SSG 20 mg/kg/day; PM 15 mg/kg/day for 17 days). The aim was to compare the efficacy and safety of PM monotherapy and the combination of SSG and PM to the reference arm of SSG alone. The primary efficacy end point was definitive cure defined as parasite clearance from splenic, bone marrow or lymph node aspirates six months after the end of treatment.

Summary of findings

In the comparison between PM monotherapy and SSG alone, 205 patients were enrolled in each arm with primary efficacy data available for 198 and 200 patients respectively. In the comparison between the SSG/PM combination and the SSG

Fig. 3.7.   **Clinical examination of a 4-year-old girl with visceral leishmaniasis (*kala-azar*), in Sudan**

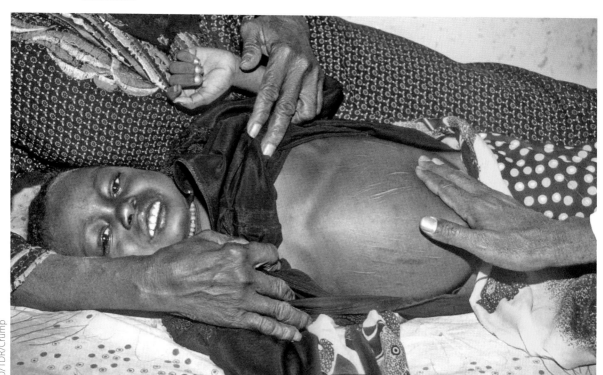

WHO/TDR/Crump

reference, 381 and 386 patients were enrolled in each arm respectively with efficacy data available for 359 patients per arm.

The efficacy of PM monotherapy was significantly lower than the efficacy observed in the SSG reference arm (84.3% versus 94.1%, difference 9.7%; 95% CI: 3.6–15.7%). The efficacy of the SSG/PM combination given for a shorter duration of 17 days was similar to the efficacy of SSG given alone for 30 days (91.4% versus 93.9%, difference 2.5%; 95% CI: 1.3–6.3%). There were no apparent differences in the safety profile of the three treatment regimens.

Towards universal health coverage

The reduced duration of treatment with the combination of SSG and PM compared to SSG alone (17 versus 30 days) reduced the treatment burden on patients and health facilities and lowered the associated costs. The cost of the drugs also favoured the combination treatment over SSG monotherapy (US $44 versus US $56). The potential risk of parasite resistance to SSG was also limited by combination therapy.

The findings supported the introduction of SSG/PM combination therapy for treatment of VL in East Africa. A WHO Expert Committee recommended its use as a first-line treatment for VL in East Africa.

Main conclusions

- The 17-day shorter duration combination treatment with SSG and PM for VL was similar in efficacy to the standard 30-day SSG treatment and had a good safety profile. Changing to this combination therapy would therefore reduce the treatment burden on patients and health facilities and limit the risk of development of drug resistance.

- The findings supported the introduction of SSG and PM combination therapy as a first-line treatment for VL in East Africa.

Case-study 8

Task shifting in the scale-up of interventions to improve child survival: an observational multicountry study in Bangladesh, Brazil, Uganda and the United Republic of Tanzania

The need for research

WHO estimates that the global health workforce has a deficit of more than four million persons (*51*). Countries with high child mortality rates also tend to have a lack of qualified health workers. The Integrated Management of Childhood Illness (IMCI) is a global strategy that has been adopted by more than 100 countries with a view to reducing child mortality. IMCI clinical guidelines describe how to assess, classify and manage children younger than five years of age who have common illnesses (*52*). One of the main barriers to expanding IMCI coverage is the lack of qualified health workers. Task shifting, which is the term used to describe the process whereby specific tasks are moved, where appropriate, to health workers with fewer qualifications and a shorter duration of pre-service training is seen as an option to address shortages of personnel (*53*).

There is a scarcity of published evaluations of the quality of clinical care provided by non-physician health workers who administer IMCI. Such evidence is needed to assess whether task shifting can be promoted as a strategy for scaling up IMCI, and for improving child health in underserved areas.

Study design

An observational multicountry study was conducted in primary government health facilities in Bangladesh, Brazil, Uganda and the United Republic of Tanzania (*11*). The clinical performance of health workers with a longer duration of pre-service training (such as doctors and clinical officers) was compared with those having a shorter duration of training (all other health workers such as nurses, midwives and nurse assistants providing clinical care). The quality of care was evaluated using standardized indicators and according to whether the assessment, classification and management of sick children by IMCI guidelines had been fully carried out. Every child was assessed twice, first by the IMCI-trained health worker who was being assessed and second by a supervisor who was blinded to the original diagnosis and treatment made by the health worker. Although this research has been classified as a study of the management of diseases and conditions, it is also health policy and systems research.

Summary of findings

The study included a total of 1262 children from 265 government health facilities: 272 children from Bangladesh, 147 from Brazil, 231 from the United Republic of Tanzania, and 612 from Uganda. In Brazil, 58% of health workers with training of long duration provided correct management, compared with 84% of those with shorter duration of training. In Uganda the figures were 23% and 33% respectively (Table 3.5). Similarly, in Bangladesh and the United Republic of Tanzania, the proportions of children managed correctly by both categories of health workers were approximately the same. Therefore, there was no evidence from any of the four settings that a shorter duration of training compromised the quality of child care.

One important caveat is that both categories of health workers performed poorly (e.g. "children correctly managed") in Uganda. The reasons for the poor performance are unknown.

Table 3.5. **Assessment, classification and management of children by IMCI-trained health workers, classified by length of pre-service training**

	Longer duration of training	Shorter duration of training
Index of assessment of children[a]		
Bangladesh	0.73	0.72
Brazil	0.48	0.53
Uganda	0.59	0.60
United Republic of Tanzania	0.94	0.88
Children correctly classified[b]		
Bangladesh	0.72	0.67
Brazil	0.61	0.73
Uganda	0.45	0.39
United Republic of Tanzania	0.76	0.80
Children correctly managed[c]		
Bangladesh	0.63	0.68
Brazil	0.58	0.84
Uganda	0.23	0.33
United Republic of Tanzania	0.64	0.63

IMCI, integrated management of childhood illness.

[a] This index assesses the quality and completeness of the clinical assessment provided to sick children based on 17 standardized items (e.g. check for fever, diarrhoea etc).

[b] Classification of diseases based on IMCI Guidelines.

[c] Correct management based on IMCI Guidelines.

Adapted, by permission of the publisher, from Huicho et al. (*11*).

It should also be noted that these assessments were made at the primary care level where fewer children have serious illnesses (the proportion of hospital referrals ranged from 1% in Brazil to 13% in Uganda). Furthermore, health workers with a shorter duration of training may be more willing to comply with standard clinical guidelines (and therefore be judged to have managed children correctly) whereas those with longer training may use a wider variety of different procedures and yet obtain equally good outcomes. In addition, the age of health workers and years of practice were not taken into consideration, both of which may compensate for duration of training.

Towards universal health coverage

These findings suggest that IMCI can be implemented by non-physician health workers who have had relatively short periods of pre-service training. Although all cadres of health workers apparently need additional training in some settings, task shifting has the potential to expand the capacity of IMCI and other child survival interventions in underserved areas faced with staff shortages (*54–56*). Randomized trials have also shown that task shifting from doctors to other less qualified health workers is possible and can be beneficial where health service staff are in short supply (*57–59*).

Main conclusions

- Task shifting from health workers with longer duration of training (doctors, clinical officers) to those with shorter duration of training (nurses, midwives and nurse assistants) did not compromise the quality of child care provided as part of IMCI.

- Task shifting could be used to increase the coverage of IMCI and other child survival interventions in underserved areas faced with staff shortages, although additional training may be needed in some settings.

Case-study 9

Improving access to emergency obstetric care: an operational research study in rural Burundi

The need for research

MDG 5 sets the target of reducing the maternal mortality ratio (MMR) by 75% between 1990 and 2015. The MMR is an important measure of maternal health at the population level and is defined as the number of maternal deaths in a given time period per 100 000 live births during the same time period (60). Although maternal mortality decreased in low- and middle-income countries from 440 deaths per 100 000 live births in 1990 to 290 per 100 000 in 2008, this 34% reduction is well short of the 75% target set for the MDG for 2015, which at the current pace would seem unachievable (61). The MMR in Burundi is among the highest in the world at 800 per 100 000 live births (in comparison, Sweden has a ratio of two per 100 000 live births) (62).

Although access to an emergency obstetric care (EMOC) package is a widely accepted intervention for reducing maternal deaths, no published data exist from Africa that quantify the population-level impact of improving availability and access to such care. Would the provision of a centralized EMOC facility, coupled with an effective patient referral and transfer system for obstetric complications, in a rural district substantially and rapidly reduce maternal deaths in order that the MDG target is achieved?

Study design

A retrospective cohort study estimated the impact of establishing a centralized EMOC facility and an ambulance transfer system on the reduction of maternal mortality in relation to MDG 5 in Kabezi district of rural Burundi (12). All nine peripheral health centre maternity units in the district were linked to a central EMOC facility and an ambulance service via cell phones or high frequency radios. On receiving a woman with an obstetric complication, health centre staff contacted the EMOC facility and an ambulance was dispatched (accompanied by a trained midwife) to transfer the woman to the EMOC facility. The distance from health centres to the EMOC facility ranged from 1 km to 70 km.

The impact of the intervention was calculated by estimating how many deaths were averted among women with a severe acute maternal morbidity (SAMM) who were transferred to and treated at the EMOC facility. This was derived by comparing the number of deaths among women with SAMM who were beneficiaries of the EMOC intervention with the expected number of deaths among the same group of women assuming that the EMOC intervention had not existed (63). SAMM was defined in terms of a specific set of conditions, including prolonged or obstructed labour requiring a caesarean section or instrumental (vacuum-assisted) delivery, complicated abortion (spontaneous or induced), pre-eclampsia/eclampsia, and prepartum or postpartum haemorrhage (Table 3.6). Using the estimate of averted deaths, the resulting theoretical MMR in Kabezi was calculated and compared to the MDG 5 target for Burundi.

Summary of findings

During 2011, 1385 women were transferred to the EMOC facility, of whom 765 (55%) had a SAMM condition (Table 3.6). The intervention package averted an estimated 74% (95% CI: 55–99%) of maternal deaths in the district, equivalent to a

Table 3.6. **Emergency obstetric complications and interventions classified as severe acute maternal morbidity (SAMM), Kabezi, Burundi, 2011**

Emergency	No (%)
Total	765 (100)
Prolonged/obstructed labour requiring caesarean section or instrumental delivery	267 (35)
Complicated abortion (spontaneous or induced)	226 (30)
Prepartum or postpartum haemorrhage	91 (12)
Caesarean section due to excessively elevated uterus or abnormal presentation of the baby requiring caesarean section	73 (10)
Dead baby in utero with uterine contractions > 48 hours	46 (6)
Pre-eclampsia	18 (2)
Sepsis	15 (2)
Uterine rupture	14 (2)
Ectopic pregnancy	5 (0.7)
Malaria	4 (0.5)
Severe anaemia	4 (0.5)
Emergency hysterectomy	2 (0.3)

Adapted, by permission of the publisher, from Tayler-Smith et al. (*12*).

Fig. 3.8. **Estimated maternal mortality ratio in Kabezi, Burundi**

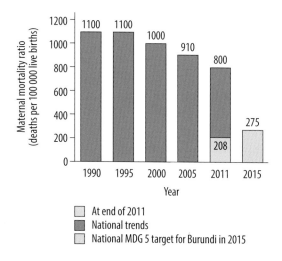

At end of 2011
National trends
National MDG 5 target for Burundi in 2015

MDG, Millennium Development Goal.
Note: maternal mortality ratio was 208.
Reproduced, by permission of the publisher, from Tayler-Smith et al. (*12*).

district MMR of 208 (95% CI: 8–360) deaths per 100 000 live births. This MMR was within the range of the 2015 MDG 5 target for Burundi (275 deaths per 100 000 live births) and was achieved well before the scheduled 2015 target (Fig. 3.8).

A potential limitation of the study is that women were diagnosed with a SAMM on the basis of clinical acumen, and this may have influenced the number of SAMM cases. However, standard case definitions for SAMM were available and clinicians were well trained in their use, and this should have limited any error in estimates.

Towards universal health coverage

The findings indicate that the provision of EMOC, combined with a functional patient referral transfer system, can markedly reduce maternal mortality. This is one way of making progress towards universal health coverage, and towards MDG 5 in rural Africa. The challenge ahead is to ensure that funds and other resources are available to scale up and sustain the achievements to 2015 and beyond. Further research is needed on cost–effectiveness and how to adapt such interventions to different settings.

Main conclusions

- The provision of a facility for EMOC, coupled with a functional ambulance transfer system for patients, was associated with a rapid and substantial reduction in maternal mortality.

- This is one example of improved health care – an intervention by which Burundi and other countries can make progress towards universal health coverage and towards the target set for MDG 5.

Case-study 10

Conditional cash transfers to improve the use of health services and health outcomes: a systematic review of evidence from low- and middle-income countries

The need for research

Conditional cash transfers (CCTs) provide payments to households on the condition that they comply with certain predetermined requirements in relation to health care or other social programmes (Fig. 3.9). CCT programmes have been justified on the basis that providing subsidies is necessary to encourage the use of and access to health services by poor people (64).

CCT schemes are intended as a financial incentive for people to adopt healthy behaviours, and to increase the demand for and utilization of health services by reducing or eliminating financial barriers to access. What is the evidence that such an approach works?

Study design

A systematic review assessed the available evidence on effectiveness of CCTs in improving access to care (utilization of health services) and

health outcomes, particularly for poorer populations in low- and middle-income countries (13). Studies from Brazil, Colombia, Honduras, Malawi, Mexico and Nicaragua were included.

Summary of findings

In terms of utilization of health services, CCT was associated with a 27% increase in individuals taking up HIV testing (one study, Malawi), an 11–20% increase in children attending health centres in the previous month, and 23–33% more children under four years of age attending preventive health-care visits. In terms of anthropometric outcomes, positive effects were found on child growth, including an increase in height of about 1 cm among children up to four years of age and a decrease in the probability of being stunted, underweight or chronically malnourished. With regard to other health outcomes, mothers reported a 20–25% decrease in the probability of children under three years of age being ill in the previous month.

Further recent evidence on the effect of CCTs has come from a randomized controlled trial in rural Malawi, which assessed the effect of cash payments in reducing HIV risk in young women (65). Schoolgirls and young women aged 13–22 years were randomly allocated monthly cash payments or nothing at all. Those receiving monthly cash payments were further subdivided into two groups: those who received the payments conditionally (on attending school for 80% of the days that the school was in session during the previous month) or unconditionally (simply by going to the cash transfer points). Households received varied amounts of US$ 4–10 and the amount given to the girl varied in the range US$ 1–5. Among the 1289 schoolgirls enrolled, HIV prevalence 18 months after enrolment was 1.2% in the cash transfer group and 3.0% in the control group (odds ratio 0.36; 95% CI: 0.14–0.91). The prevalence of herpes simplex virus type 2 (HSV-2) was 0.7% in the cash transfer group and 3.0% in the control group (odds ratio 0.24; 95% CI: 0.09–0.65). There were no

Fig. 3.9. **Identity cards are an integral part of schemes that provide conditional cash transfers in health and education programmes**

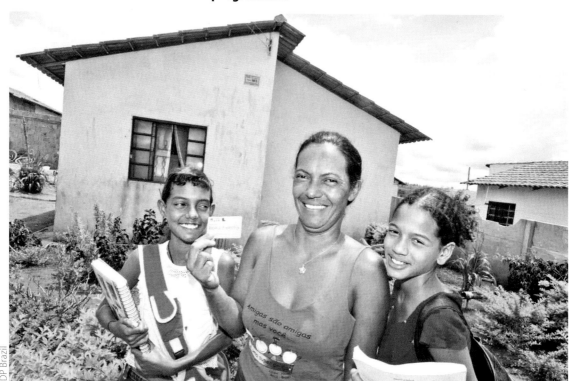

UNDP Brazil

differences between the conditional and unconditional cash transfer groups in HIV or HSV-2 prevalence. These findings show that financially empowering schoolgirls might have a beneficial effect on their sexual and reproductive health.

In Brazil, a country-wide ecological study showed that increased coverage of the *Bolsa Familia* programme, a national CCT programme transferring cash to poor households if they comply with conditions related to health and education, was significantly associated with the reduction of mortality (whether from all causes or from poverty-related causes) in children under five years of age. The effect of consolidated *Bolsa Familia* coverage was highest on mortality resulting from malnutrition and diarrhoea

in the under-fives. In addition, the programme was shown to increase vaccination coverage and prenatal visits by mothers and to reduce hospitalization rates in the under-fives (66).

Towards universal health coverage

There is now a substantial body of data showing that CCTs can, under some circumstances, have positive effects on nutritional status and health by increasing the use of health services and by promoting healthy behaviours (13, 67–69). However, CCT schemes do not necessarily work everywhere. Their success depends on a variety of factors, such as being able to identify participating individuals with unique person identifiers (Fig. 3.9), and on having effective and reliable mechanisms to disburse payments. There are also limitations to the studies that have been carried out to date. For instance, trials that demonstrate changes in short-term behaviour do not guarantee changes in long-term attitudes to health. It is clearly important to find the right mix of incentives and regulations that affect both the supply of and demand for services so that CCTs can improve the quality of care in any given setting (*68*). This is a goal for further research.

Main conclusions

- CCT schemes serve as financial incentives for increasing the demand for and utilization of health services by reducing or eliminating financial barriers to access.
- Studies from several low- and middle-income countries show that CCT schemes can, in some circumstances, increase health service utilization which leads to improved health outcomes.

Case-study 11

Insurance in the provision of accessible and affordable health services: a randomized controlled trial in Mexico

The need for research

In 2003, Mexico initiated a new set of health reforms which aimed to provide health coverage to approximately 50 million people who were without any form of financial protection for health. Before 2003, the right to health care was an employment benefit that was restricted to the salaried workforce. A large majority of the poor population was non-salaried or unemployed, and a significant proportion was at risk of catastrophic or impoverishing health expenditure.

The 2003 Mexican health reform legislated the System of Social Protection in Health, of which *Seguro Popular* (People's insurance) was the new public insurance scheme that assures legislated access to comprehensive health care. In the first few years of *Seguro Popular*, and taking advantage of its phased roll-out, it was important to assess the impact of the intervention on health and financial expenditure (*70*).

Study design

In a cluster randomized study, 100 pairs of health facility catchment areas ("health clusters") were randomly assigned to receive either the intervention or the control. The intervention, *Seguro Popular*, provided a package of benefits that included coverage for 266 health interventions and 312 medicines, and increased funds to state health ministries proportional to the number of families joining the scheme. There were also funds to cover catastrophic health expenditures associated with certain diseases. In health clusters receiving the intervention, there was a campaign to persuade every family to enrol in *Seguro Popular*. In the matched control cluster families received the usual health care which they had to pay for (*14*). The main outcomes were details of expenditures which were classified as out-of-pocket expenditures for all health services, while catastrophic expenditures were defined as health spending greater than 30% of capacity to pay (measured in terms of income).

Summary of findings

In the intervention clusters, out-of-pocket expenses and catastrophic expenditures were 23% lower than in the control clusters. Among those households within intervention clusters that signed up to *Seguro Popular* (44% on average), catastrophic expenditures were reduced by 59%. Among persons enrolled in the *Seguro Popular* programme, 69% rated the quality of health services as very good or good, and 85% reported that the programme benefits were explained clearly by programme officials. Surprisingly, and contrary to previous observational studies, there was no substantial effect of *Seguro Popular* on the quality of care (such as improving access to and use of medical facilities or reducing drug stock-outs) or on increasing coverage for chronic illness. These findings might be explained by the short assessment period of 10 months (*71, 72*). Although these results are encouraging, further research is needed to ascertain the long-term effects of the programme.

Towards universal health coverage

The project design for assessing the effects of *Seguro Popular* proved robust and showed that the programme did indeed reach the poor. In August 2012, within 10 years of launching the scheme, 52 million previously uninsured Mexicans had state-protected health care. Taking into account coverage with a range of insurance schemes, approximately 98% of 113 million people in Mexico had financial risk protection in 2012, and Mexico has celebrated the achievement of universal health coverage (*70, 73*). Nevertheless, further experimental research is needed with a longer period of follow-up in order to measure the effects on access to, and use of, health facilities and health outcomes. This needs to be done not only in Mexico but also in other countries planning public health policy reforms.

Main conclusions

- In Mexico, implementation of a public national health insurance scheme, *Seguro Popular*, led to the country celebrating universal health coverage less than 10 years after its introduction.
- *Seguro Popular* resulted in a 23% reduction in out-of-pocket expenses and catastrophic expenditures, with benefits reaching poorer households.
- Such insurance schemes have the potential to contribute to the achievement of universal health coverage in other countries.

Case-study 12

Affordable health care in ageing populations: forecasting changes in public health expenditure in five European countries

The need for research

As the average age of European populations becomes older, a larger number of people will suffer from chronic disease and disability as a result of cancers, cardiovascular diseases, fractures, dementia and other conditions. In addition, a growing number of people will suffer from several morbidities at the same time. These observations have generated concern that public spending on health care in ageing populations will become unaffordable.

Study design

Using published data on forecasts of population ageing, and on current health expenditure by age, Rechel and co-workers calculated the expected annual changes in per capita health expenditure associated with ageing over the period 2010–2060 (*74*). They assumed that health expenditure per person in each age group would be constant over the 50-year period, and that the unit costs of health care would also remain unchanged. The analysis was carried out for five countries of the European Union (EU) – the Czech Republic, Germany, Hungary, the Netherlands and Slovenia.

Summary of findings

The projected increases in health expenditure associated with ageing were modest. The annual increases in per capita expenditure, calculated as means for five-year periods, were consistent across the five countries. They were never more than 1% of the mean annual expenditure, and they declined from the 2030s onwards (Fig. 3.10). In the Netherlands, for example, the increase in spending per person is expected to peak between 2020 and

Fig. 3.10.   Projected changes in per capita public health expenditure associated with ageing in five European countries, 2010–2060

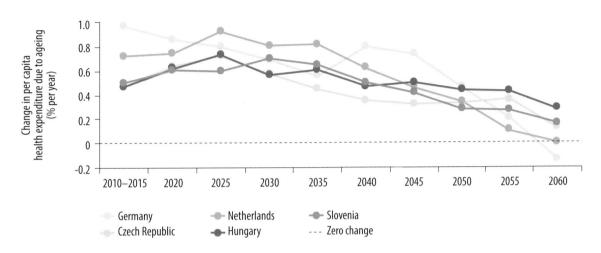

Note: Points are annual average percentage increases, calculated as five-year means, derived from data on projected population ageing and on current patterns of health expenditure by age.
Reproduced, by permission of the publisher, from Rechel et al. (74).

2025, resulting in an average yearly growth rate of 0.9% due to ageing, falling to zero between 2055 and 2060, when the population of the Netherlands is likely to become younger on average.

Towards universal health coverage

The common assumption that population ageing will drive future health expenditure to unaffordable levels is not supported by this analysis. These results are in line with some other assessments which have found that ageing is not expected to incur substantial increases in health-care costs (83). A study carried out for the European Commission forecast moderate increases in public-sector health spending due to ageing in the EU, growing from 6.7% of GDP in 2007 to 8.2% in 2060 (84). If, with increases in life expectancy, the proportion of life in good health does not change, then public expenditure on health care is expected to increase by only 0.7%, to 7.4% of GDP.

Research on the cost of dying shows that the proximity of death is a more important predictor of high health-care expenditure than is ageing (85, 86). A large proportion of lifetime expenditure on health-care typically occurs in the last year of life, particularly in the last few weeks before death (87), and health-care expenditure tends to be lower for those who are most elderly (> 80 years). Furthermore, although older people are major consumers of health care, other factors – notably technological developments – have a greater effect on total health care costs (74).

Nevertheless, the growing proportion of older people in European populations does present some challenges for health and welfare if, for instance, a declining fraction of the population has to bear the rising costs of health and social care and pensions. Yet these challenges are not insuperable. The measures that can be taken include: promoting good health throughout life, thereby increasing the chance that additional years of life are spent in good health; minimizing the severity of chronic disease through early detection and care; improving the efficiency of health systems so they are better able to cope with the needs of older people; and increasing the participation of older people in the labour force (*74, 88*).

Main conclusions

- Between 2010 and 2060, the estimated annual increases in health expenditure due to ageing are less than 1% and falling in five European countries.
- While the number of older people suffering chronic diseases and disability is expected to grow, the costs of health care become substantial only in the last year of life.
- Although ageing is not expected to incur large extra costs, systems for health care, long-term social care and welfare in European countries must adapt to population ageing.

Conclusions: general lessons drawn from specific examples

The 12 case-studies presented in this chapter, ranging from the control of malaria to the provision of health insurance, are examples of research that illuminate the path to universal health coverage. They address a diversity of questions about reaching universal coverage. They employ a range of research methods – quantitative and qualitative evaluations, observational and case–control studies, non-randomized intervention studies, randomized controlled trials, and systematic reviews and meta-analyses. They show the potential benefits of having evidence from multiple sources, and explore the link between experimental design and strength of inference. They reveal the nature of the research cycle in which questions lead to answers which lead to yet more questions. And they show how research works at the interface with policy and practice.

Six features of these case-studies deserve emphasis. First, the most appropriate research methods – those that find the best compromise between cost, time and validity – vary along the research cycle. In general, randomized controlled trials and trials using a minimization method for allocation give the most robust answers to questions about the efficacy of an intervention, provided they have been assessed to be valid by rigorous critical appraisal. However, judging the effectiveness of interventions during routine practice is more difficult because there are no experimental controls (*75, 76*). Nevertheless, operational questions relating to staffing needs, infrastructure and commodity supply chains can often be answered by a process of "learning by doing" – i.e. by practice and repetition, correcting errors and making improvements after evaluation, usually with minor innovations. This appears to be the dominant method of addressing health insurance reforms in Africa and Asia, but whether uncontrolled interventions (i.e. those not tested by a formal experiment) lead to the best outcomes is open to debate (*77*).

In the face of health emergencies, some experimental designs carry the disadvantage of being costly, slow and logistically complex, whereas observational studies can be done quickly and cheaply – yet are potentially at risk of giving misleading conclusions. However, there are instances in which that risk is worth taking and results in positive outcomes. In responding to the enormous demand for antiretroviral therapy for HIV/AIDS in sub-Saharan Africa, observational research on task shifting and on the decentralization of health services yielded important data that could inform policy and practice before evidence became available from controlled experiments (*78, 79*). However, recent successful efforts to modify and apply formal experimental designs (especially randomized designs) for use beyond clinical trials (e.g. to address problems of health service access and delivery) suggest that experimental rigour need not always be sacrificed for the sake of obtaining results rapidly and cheaply (*80*).

Second, the continuous cycle of asking and answering questions implies that the implementation of research solutions (the best answers at any given moment) can be effectively monitored. However, the current metrics used to judge the success of new interventions, and the systems for collecting the relevant data, are far from adequate (*81*).

Third, the goal of this report is to promote research that makes the coverage of health interventions truly universal. Access to health services cannot be the privilege of those who live in relatively peaceful areas of the world. In 2009 alone, there were 31 armed conflicts worldwide (*82*). These circumstances demand imaginative methods for the provision of health care. In this context, telemedicine is an example of an enabling technology (Case-study 4).

Fourth, while some of the case-studies in this chapter show how research can influence practice, health policy and action are not determined by evidence alone (Box 2.1). Some common reasons why research findings are not used include: the research question is not relevant to the problems faced by health workers or policy-makers; the research

findings, though published in peer-reviewed journals, are not clearly explained to those who might use them; and the solutions arising from research are too costly or too complex to implement (*81*).

Fifth, although the 12 examples in this chapter relate to a wide range of conditions of ill-health and methods for studying them, the examples inevitably leave some gaps. Some of the topics missing from this chapter are no less important than those that are covered, such as finding ways to prepare for pandemics, to mitigate environmental hazards, or to assess the health benefits of agriculture (Box 2.6).

Finally, the examples in this chapter point to the advantages of creating a structured system for carrying out research in low- and middle-income countries, and of deepening the culture of enquiry in every setting where research is carried out. To advance this cause, Chapter 4 describes the architecture of systems that can effectively carry out research for universal health coverage. ■

References

1. UK Clinical Research Collaboration. *Health research classification system*. London, Medical Research Council, 2009. (http://www.hrcsonline.net/, accessed 17 March 2013).
2. *Health research classification systems – current approaches and future recommendations*. Strasbourg, European Science Foundation, 2011.
3. Lim SS et al. Net benefits: a multicountry analysis of observational data examining associations between insecticide-treated mosquito nets and health outcomes. *PLoS Medicine*, 2011,8:e1001091. doi: http://dx.doi.org/10.1371/journal.pmed.1001091 PMID:21909249
4. Eisele TP, Steketee RW. African malaria control programs deliver ITNs and achieve what the clinical trials predicted. *PLoS Medicine*, 2011,8:e1001088. doi: http://dx.doi.org/10.1371/journal.pmed.1001088 PMID:21909247
5. Cohen MS et al. Prevention of HIV-1 infection with early antiretroviral therapy. *The New England Journal of Medicine*, 2011,365:493-505. doi: http://dx.doi.org/10.1056/NEJMoa1105243 PMID:21767103
6. Brooks WA et al. Effect of weekly zinc supplements on incidence of pneumonia and diarrhoea in children younger than 2 years in an urban, low-income population in Bangladesh: randomised controlled trial. *Lancet*, 2005,366:999-1004. doi: http://dx.doi.org/10.1016/S0140-6736(05)67109-7 PMID:16168782
7. Zachariah R et al. Practicing medicine without borders: tele-consultations and tele-mentoring for improving paediatric care in a conflict setting in Somalia? *Tropical Medicine & International Health*, 2012,17:1156-1162. doi: http://dx.doi.org/10.1111/j.1365-3156.2012.03047.x PMID:22845678
8. Boehme CC et al. Rapid molecular detection of tuberculosis and rifampin resistance. *The New England Journal of Medicine*, 2010,363:1005-1015. doi: http://dx.doi.org/10.1056/NEJMoa0907847 PMID:20825313
9. Yusuf S et al. Effects of a polypill (Polycap) on risk factors in middle-aged individuals without cardiovascular disease (Trends Pharmacol Sci): a phase II, double-blind, randomised trial. *Lancet*, 2009,373:1341-1351. doi: http://dx.doi.org/10.1016/S0140-6736(09)60611-5 PMID:19339045

10. Musa A et al. Sodium stibogluconate (SSG) & paromomycin combination compared to SSG for visceral leishmaniasis in East Africa: a randomised controlled trial. *PLoS neglected tropical diseases*, 2012,6:e1674. doi: http://dx.doi.org/10.1371/journal.pntd.0001674 PMID:22724029

11. Huicho L et al. How much does quality of child care vary between health workers with differing durations of training? An observational multicountry study. *Lancet*, 2008,372:910-916. doi: http://dx.doi.org/10.1016/S0140-6736(08)61401-4 PMID:18790314

12. Tayler-Smith K et al. Achieving the Millennium Development Goal of reducing maternal mortality in rural Africa: an experience from Burundi. *Tropical Medicine & International Health*, 2013,18:166-174. doi: http://dx.doi.org/10.1111/tmi.12022 PMID:23163431

13. Lagarde M, Haines A, Palmer N. The impact of conditional cash transfers on health outcomes and use of health services in low and middle income countries. *Cochrane database of systematic reviews (Online)*,, 2009,4:CD008137. PMID:19821444

14. King G et al. Public policy for the poor? A randomised assessment of the Mexican universal health insurance programme. *Lancet*, 2009,373:1447-1454. doi: http://dx.doi.org/10.1016/S0140-6736(09)60239-7 PMID:19359034

15. Lienhardt C, Cobelens FG. Operational research for improved tuberculosis control: the scope, the needs and the way forward. *The International Journal of Tuberculosis and Lung Disease*, 2011,15:6-13. PMID:21276290

16. Nachega JB et al. Current status and future prospects of epidemiology and public health training and research in the WHO African region. *International Journal of Epidemiology*, 2012,41:1829-1846. doi: http://dx.doi.org/10.1093/ije/dys189 PMID:23283719

17. Eisele TP, Larsen D, Steketee RW. Protective efficacy of interventions for preventing malaria mortality in children in Plasmodium falciparum endemic areas. *International Journal of Epidemiology*, 2010,39:Suppl 1:i88-i101. doi: http://dx.doi.org/10.1093/ije/dyq026 PMID:20348132

18. Lengeler C. Insecticide-treated bednets and curtains for preventing malaria. *Cochrane Database of Systematic Reviews (Online)*, 2000,2CD000363. PMID:10796535

19. Flaxman AD et al. Rapid scaling up of insecticide-treated bed net coverage in Africa and its relationship with development assistance for health: a systematic synthesis of supply, distribution, and household survey data. *PLoS Medicine*, 2010,7:e1000328. doi: http://dx.doi.org/10.1371/journal.pmed.1000328 PMID:20808957

20. *Malaria funding and resource utilization: the first decade of Roll Back Malaria*. Geneva, World Health Organization on behalf of the Roll Back Malaria Partnership, 2010.

21. Eisele TP, Steketee RW. Distribution of insecticide treated nets in rural Africa. *BMJ (Clinical research Ed.)*, 2009,339:b1598. doi: http://dx.doi.org/10.1136/bmj.b1598 PMID:19574313

22. *UNAIDS report on the global AIDS epidemic 2012*. Geneva, Joint United Nations Programme on HIV/AIDS, 2012.

23. Alberts B. Science breakthroughs. *Science*, 2011,334:1604. doi: http://dx.doi.org/10.1126/science.1217831 PMID:22194530

24. *Guidance on couples HIV testing and counselling including antiretroviral therapy for treatment and prevention in serodiscordant couples. Recommendations for a public health approach*. Geneva, World Health Organization, 2012.

25. Schouten EJ et al. Prevention of mother-to-child transmission of HIV and the health-related Millennium Development Goals: time for a public health approach. *Lancet*, 2011,378:282-284. doi: http://dx.doi.org/10.1016/S0140-6736(10)62303-3 PMID:21763940

26. *Programmatic update. Use of antiretroviral drugs for treating pregnant women and preventing HIV infection in infants*. Geneva, World Health Organization, 2012.

27. Caulfield LE, Black RE. Zinc deficiency. In: Ezzati M et al., eds. *Comparative quantification of health risks: Global and regional burden of disease attribution to selected major risk factors*. Geneva, World Health Organization, 2004:257–279.

28. Bhutta ZA et al. Therapeutic effects of oral zinc in acute and persistent diarrhea in children in developing countries: pooled analysis of randomized controlled trials. *The American Journal of Clinical Nutrition*, 2000,72:1516-1522. PMID:11101480

29. Bhutta ZA et al. Prevention of diarrhea and pneumonia by zinc supplementation in children in developing countries: pooled analysis of randomized controlled trials. Zinc Investigators' Collaborative Group. *The Journal of Pediatrics*, 1999,135:689-697. doi: http://dx.doi.org/10.1016/S0022-3476(99)70086-7 PMID:10586170

30. *Joint statement. Clinical management of acute diarrhoea*. New York, NY, United Nations Children's Fund and Geneva, World Health Organization, 2004.

31. Sood S et al. What is telemedicine? A collection of 104 peer-reviewed perspectives and theoretical underpinnings. *Telemedicine Journal and e-Health*, 2007,13:573-590. doi: http://dx.doi.org/10.1089/tmj.2006.0073 PMID:17999619

32. Spooner SA, Gotlieb EM. Telemedicine: pediatric applications. *Pediatrics*, 2004,113:e639-e643. doi: http://dx.doi.org/10.1542/peds.113.6.e639 PMID:15173548

33. Wootton R, Bonnardot L. In what circumstances is telemedicine appropriate in the developing world? *JRSM Short Reports*, 2010,1:37. doi: http://dx.doi.org/10.1258/shorts.2010.010045 PMID:21103129

34. Shiferaw F, Zolfo M. The role of information communication technology (ICT) towards universal health coverage: the first steps of a telemedicine project in Ethiopia. *Global Health Action*, 2012,5:1-8. doi: http://dx.doi.org/10.3402/gha.v5i0.15638 PMID:22479235

35. Coulborn RM et al. Feasibility of using teleradiology to improve tuberculosis screening and case management in a district hospital in Malawi. *Bulletin of the World Health Organization*, 2012,90:705-711. doi: http://dx.doi.org/10.2471/BLT.11.099473 PMID:22984316

36. *Global tuberculosis report2012*. Geneva, World Health Organization, 2012.

37. *Automated real-time nucleic acid amplification technology for rapid and simultaneous detection of tuberculosis and rifampicin resistance: Xpert MTB/RIF system. Policy statement*. Geneva, World Health Organization, 2011.

38. Weyer K et al. Rapid molecular TB diagnosis: evidence, policy-making and global implementation of Xpert®MTB/RIF. *The European Respiratory Journal*, 2012, doi: http://dx.doi.org/10.1183/09031936.00157212 PMID:23180585

39. WHO monitoring of Xpert MTB/RIF roll-out (web site). Geneva, World Health Organization, 2012. (http://who.int/tb/laboratory/mtbrifrollout, accessed 17 March 2013).

40. Boehme CC et al. Feasibility, diagnostic accuracy, and effectiveness of decentralised use of the Xpert MTB/RIF test for diagnosis of tuberculosis and multidrug resistance: a multicentre implementation study. *Lancet*, 2011,377:1495-1505. doi: http://dx.doi.org/10.1016/S0140-6736(11)60438-8 PMID:21507477

41. Pantoja A et al. Xpert MTB/RIF for diagnosis of TB and drug-resistant TB: a cost and affordability analysis. *The European Respiratory Journal*, 2012,(Epub ahead of print) doi: http://dx.doi.org/10.1183/09031936.00147912 PMID:23258774

42. *A comprehensive global monitoring framework, including indicators, and a set of voluntary global targets for the prevention and control of noncommunicable diseases*. Geneva, World Health Organization, 2012. (http://www.who.int/nmh/events/2012/discussion_paper3.pdf, accessed 17 March 2013).

43. Beaglehole R et al. Measuring progress on NCDs: one goal and five targets. *Lancet*, 2012,380:1283-1285. doi: http://dx.doi.org/10.1016/S0140-6736(12)61692-4 PMID:23063272

44. Wald NJ, Law MR. A strategy to reduce cardiovascular disease by more than 80%. *BMJ (Clinical Research Ed.)*, 2003,326:1419. doi: http://dx.doi.org/10.1136/bmj.326.7404.1419 PMID:12829553

45. Rodgers A et al. An international randomised placebo-controlled trial of a four-component combination pill ("polypill") in people with raised cardiovascular risk. *PLoS ONE*, 2011,6:e19857. doi: http://dx.doi.org/10.1371/journal.pone.0019857 PMID:21647425

46. Thom S et al. Use of a Multidrug Pill In Reducing cardiovascular Events (UMPIRE): rationale and design of a randomised controlled trial of a cardiovascular preventive polypill-based strategy in India and Europe. *European Journal of Preventive Cardiology*, 2012, doi: http://dx.doi.org/10.1177/2047487312463278

47. *Control of the leishmaniases. Report of a meeting of the WHO Expert Committee on the Control of Leishmaniases, 22–26 March 2010*. Geneva, World Health Organization, 2010 (WHO Technical Report Series, No. 949).

48. Reithinger R, Brooker S, Kolaczinski JH. Visceral leishmaniasis in eastern Africa — current status. *Transactions of the Royal Society of Tropical Medicine and Hygiene*, 2007,101:1169-1170. doi: http://dx.doi.org/10.1016/j.trstmh.2007.06.001 PMID:17632193

49. Sundar S et al. Injectable paromomycin for Visceral leishmaniasis in India. *The New England Journal of Medicine*, 2007,356:2571-2581. doi: http://dx.doi.org/10.1056/NEJMoa066536 PMID:17582067

50. Melaku Y et al. Treatment of kala-azar in southern Sudan using a 17-day regimen of sodium stibogluconate combined with paromomycin: a retrospective comparison with 30-day sodium stibogluconate monotherapy. *The American Journal of Tropical Medicine and Hygiene*, 2007,77:89-94. PMID:17620635

51. *The world health report 2006– working together for health*. Geneva, World Health Organization, 2006.

52. Gove S. Integrated management of childhood illness by outpatient health workers: technical basis and overview. The WHO Working Group on Guidelines for Integrated Management of the Sick Child. *Bulletin of the World Health Organization*, 1997,75:Suppl 17-24. PMID:9529714

53. *Task shifting. Global recommendations and guidelines*. Geneva, World Health Organization, 2008.

54. Lewin S et al. Lay health workers in primary and community health care for maternal and child health and the management of infectious diseases. *Cochrane Database of Systematic Reviews (Online)*, 2010,3CD004015. PMID:20238326

55. Ellis M et al. Intrapartum-related stillbirths and neonatal deaths in rural Bangladesh: a prospective, community-based cohort study. *Pediatrics*, 2011,127:e1182-e1190. doi: http://dx.doi.org/10.1542/peds.2010-0842 PMID:21502233

56. *WHO recommendations: optimizing health worker roles to improve access to key maternal and newborn health interventions through task shifting*. Geneva, World Health Organization, 2012.

57. Jaffar S et al. Rates of virological failure in patients treated in a home-based versus a facility-based HIV-care model in Jinja, southeast Uganda: a cluster-randomised equivalence trial. *Lancet*, 2009,374:2080-2089. doi: http://dx.doi.org/10.1016/S0140-6736(09)61674-3 PMID:19939445

58. Fairall L et al. Task shifting of antiretroviral treatment from doctors to primary-care nurses in South Africa (STRETCH): a pragmatic, parallel, cluster-randomised trial. *Lancet*, 2012,380:889-898. doi: http://dx.doi.org/10.1016/S0140-6736(12)60730-2 PMID:22901955

59. Mugyenyi P et al. Routine versus clinically driven laboratory monitoring of HIV antiretroviral therapy in Africa (DART): a randomised non-inferiority trial. *Lancet*, 2010,375:123-131. doi: http://dx.doi.org/10.1016/S0140-6736(09)62067-5 PMID:20004464

60. Graham WJ et al. Measuring maternal mortality: an overview of opportunities and options for developing countries. *BMC Medicine*, 2008,6:12. doi: http://dx.doi.org/10.1186/1741-7015-6-12 PMID:18503716

61. Maternal mortality is declining, but more needs to be done. *The Millenium Development Goal Report 2010. Addendum 2. Goal 5 Improve Maternal Health.* New York, NY, United Nations, 2010.

62. *Trends in maternal mortality: 1990–2010. WHO, UNICEF, UNFPA and The World Bank estimates.* Geneva, World Health Organization, 2012.

63. Fournier P et al. Improved access to comprehensive emergency obstetric care and its effect on institutional maternal mortality in rural Mali. *Bulletin of the World Health Organization*, 2009,87:30-38. doi: http://dx.doi.org/10.2471/BLT.07.047076 PMID:19197402

64. Oxman AD, Fretheim A. Can paying for results help to achieve the Millennium Development Goals? A critical review of selected evaluations of results-based financing. *Journal of Evidence-based Medicine*, 2009,2:184-195. doi: http://dx.doi.org/10.1111/j.1756-5391.2009.01024.x PMID:21349012

65. Baird SJ et al. Effect of a cash transfer programme for schooling on prevalence of HIV and herpes simplex type 2 in Malawi: a cluster randomised trial. *Lancet*, 2012,379:1320-1329. doi: http://dx.doi.org/10.1016/S0140-6736(11)61709-1 PMID:22341825

66. Rasella D et al. Effect of a conditional cash transfer programme on childhood mortality: a nationwide analysis of Brazilian municipalities. *Lancet*, 2013, May 14. pii:S0140-6736(13)60715-1. doi: http://dx.doi.org/10.1016/S0140-6736(13)60715-1 PMID:23683599

67. Ranganathan M, Lagarde M. Promoting healthy behaviours and improving health outcomes in low and middle income countries: a review of the impact of conditional cash transfer programmes. *Preventive Medicine*, 2012,55:Supp l:S95-S105. doi: http://dx.doi.org/10.1016/j.ypmed.2011.11.015 PMID:22178043

68. Waldman RJ, Mintz ED, Papowitz HE. The cure for cholera - improving access to safe water and sanitation. *The New England Journal of Medicine*, 2013,368:592-594. doi: http://dx.doi.org/10.1056/NEJMp1214179 PMID:23301693

69. Dye C et al. Prospects for tuberculosis elimination. *Annual Review of Public Health*, 2012 (Epub ahead of print).

70. Knaul FM et al. The quest for universal health coverage: achieving social protection for all in Mexico. *Lancet*, 2012,380:1259-1279. doi: http://dx.doi.org/10.1016/S0140-6736(12)61068-X PMID:22901864

71. Gakidou E et al. Assessing the effect of the 2001–06 Mexican health reform: an interim report card. *Lancet*, 2006,368:1920-1935. doi: http://dx.doi.org/10.1016/S0140-6736(06)69568-8 PMID:17126725

72. Hussey MA, Hughes JP. Design and analysis of stepped wedge cluster randomized trials. *Contemporary Clinical Trials*, 2007,28:182-191. doi: http://dx.doi.org/10.1016/j.cct.2006.05.007 PMID:16829207

73. Mexico: celebrating universal health coverage. *Lancet*, 2012,380:622. doi: http://dx.doi.org/10.1016/S0140-6736(12)61342-7 PMID:22901868

74. Rechel B et al. Ageing in the European Union. *Lancet*, 2013,381:1312-1322. doi: http://dx.doi.org/10.1016/S0140-6736(12)62087-X PMID:23541057

75. Glasgow RE, Lichtenstein E, Marcus AC. Why don't we see more translation of health promotion research to practice? Rethinking the efficacy-to-effectiveness transition. *American Journal of Public Health*, 2003,93:1261-1267. doi: http://dx.doi.org/10.2105/AJPH.93.8.1261 PMID:12893608

76. Sussman S et al. Translation in the health professions: converting science into action. *Evaluation & the Health Professions*, 2006,29:7-32. doi: http://dx.doi.org/10.1177/0163278705284441 PMID:16510878

77. Lagomarsino G et al. Moving towards universal health coverage: health insurance reforms in nine developing countries in Africa and Asia. *Lancet*, 2012,380:933-943. doi: http://dx.doi.org/10.1016/S0140-6736(12)61147-7 PMID:22959390

78. *Treat, train, retain. The AIDS and health workforce plan. Report on the consultation on AIDS and human resources for health.* Geneva, World Health Organization, 2006.

79. Zachariah R et al. Task shifting in HIV/AIDS: opportunities, challenges and proposed actions for sub-Saharan Africa. *Transactions of the Royal Society of Tropical Medicine and Hygiene*, 2009,103:549-558. doi: http://dx.doi.org/10.1016/j.trstmh.2008.09.019 PMID:18992905

80. Banerjee AV, Duflos E. *Poor economics*. New York, NY, Public Affairs, 2011.

81. Zachariah R et al. Is operational research delivering the goods? The journey to success in low-income countries. *The Lancet Infectious Diseases*, 2012,12:415-421. doi: http://dx.doi.org/10.1016/S1473-3099(11)70309-7 PMID:22326018

82. Armed conflicts. In: Cañadas FM et al. *Alert 2010! Report on conflicts, human rights and peacebuilding*. Barcelona, Escola de Cultura de Pau/School for a Culture of Peace, 2010. (http://www.humansecuritygateway.com/documents/ECP_Alert2010_ReportonConflictsHumanRightsandPeacebuilding.pdf, accessed 19 March 2013).

83. Figueras J, McKee M, eds. *Health systems, health, wealth and societal well-being. Assessing the case for investing in health systems*. Copenhagen, Open University Press, 2011.

84. *2009 Ageing report: economic and budgetary projections for the EU-27 Member States (2008–2060)*. Luxembourg, Office for Official Publications of the European Communities, 2009.

85. Polder JJ, Barendregt JJ, van Oers H. Health care costs in the last year of life – the Dutch experience. *Social Science & Medicine*, 2006,63:1720-1731. doi: http://dx.doi.org/10.1016/j.socscimed.2006.04.018 PMID:16781037

86. Breyer F, Felder S. Life expectancy and health care expenditures: a new calculation for Germany using the costs of dying. *Health policy (Amsterdam, Netherlands)*, 2006,75:178-186. doi: http://dx.doi.org/10.1016/j.healthpol.2005.03.011 PMID:15893848

87. Kardamanidis K et al. Hospital costs of older people in New South Wales in the last year of life. *The Medical Journal of Australia*, 2007,187:383-386. PMID:17907999

88. *Good health adds life to years. Global brief for World Health Day 2012*. Geneva, World Health Organization, 2012 (Document WHO/DCO/WHD/2012.2).

Building research systems for
universal health coverage

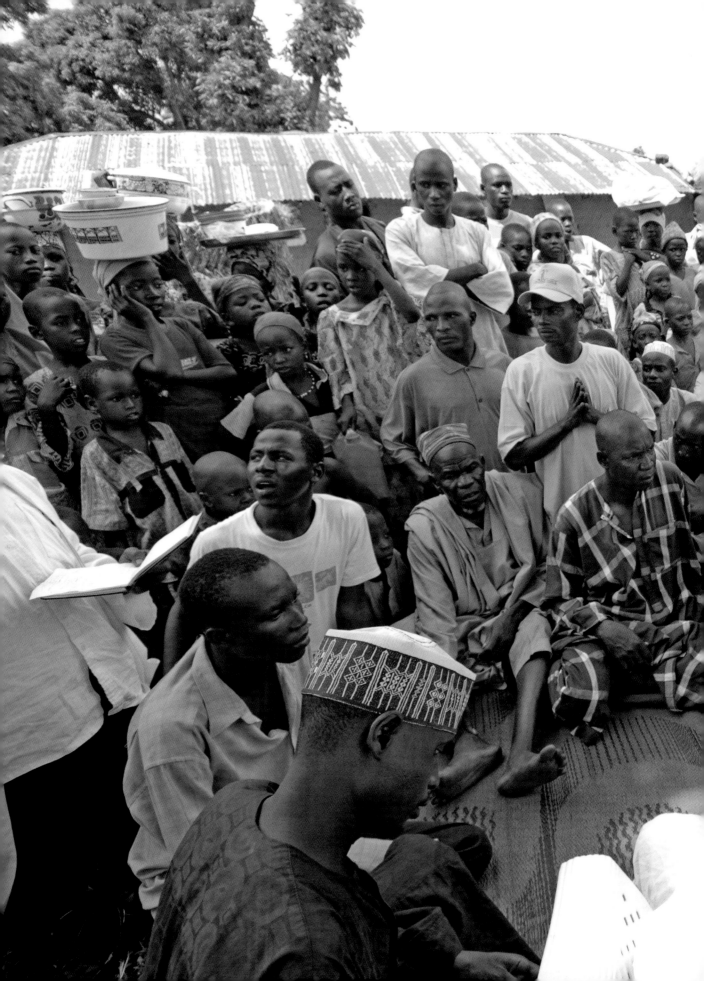

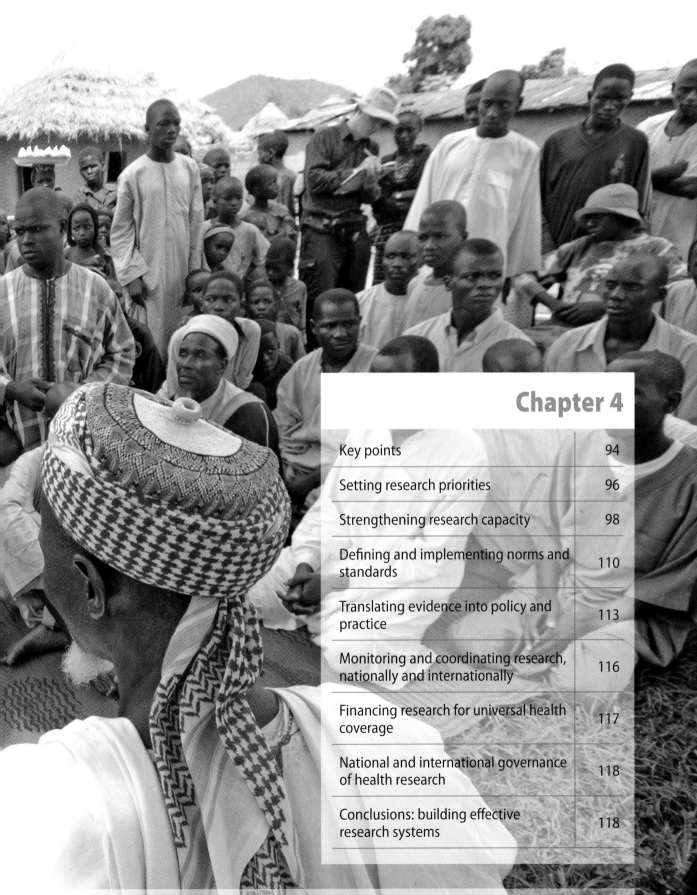

Chapter 4

Community-led management of onchocerciasis, malaria, tuberculosis and the distribution of vitamin A for infants, northern Nigeria (WHO/TDR/Andy Craggs)

Key points

- Health research systems have four essential functions: to set research priorities, to develop research capacity, to define norms and standards for research, and to translate evidence into practice. These functions support health in general and universal health coverage in particular.

- Standard methods have been developed to set research priorities, but the best-documented examples are those for specific health topics such as malaria and tuberculosis control and the reduction of child mortality. All countries should set national priorities, across all aspects of health, to determine how best to spend limited funds on research.

- Effective research needs transparent and accountable methods for allocating funds, and well-equipped research institutions and networks. However, it is the people who do research – with their curiosity, imagination, motivation, technical skills, experience and connections – who are most critical to the success of the research enterprise.

- Codes of practice, which are the cornerstone of any research system, are already in use in many countries. The task ahead is to ensure that these are comprehensive and applicable in all countries, and to encourage adherence everywhere.

- Achieving universal health coverage depends on research ranging from studies of causation to the functioning of health systems. Because many existing, cost-effective interventions are not widely used, there is a particular need to close the gap between existing knowledge and action. To help achieve that goal, research should be strengthened not only in academic centres but also in public health programmes, close to the supply of and demand for health services.

- Many of the determinants of health and disease lie outside the health system so research needs to investigate the impact of policies for "health in all sectors". Research will add to the evidence on how human activities affect health, for example through agricultural practices and changes to the natural environment.

- Mechanisms to support research include monitoring (national and international observatories), coordination (information-sharing, collaborative research studies) and financing (raising and distributing funds to support global and national research priorities).

4

Building research systems for universal health coverage

The case studies in Chapter 3 show how research can tackle some of the key questions about reaching universal health coverage. They show how research can produce results to guide policy and practice. The success of these selected studies, and of any study that aims to support universal health coverage, depends on having an environment that is conducive to doing research of the highest quality. The most credible research, reaching the largest number of people and producing the greatest benefits for health, will be done where there is an established culture of enquiry, a set of procedures for supporting and carrying out investigations, and frequent dialogue between researchers and policy-makers.

An effective health research system needs to carry out four functions in particular. It must define research questions and priorities; raise funds and develop research staff capacity and infrastructure; establish norms and standards for research practice; and translate research findings into a form that can guide policy. All four of these functions are embraced by the WHO Strategy on Research for Health (Box 4.1). Effective research systems allow investigators to go all the way round the research cycle: measuring the size of the health problem; understanding its cause(s); devising solutions; translating the evidence into policy, practice and products; and evaluating effectiveness after implementation (Box 2.3).

There are few assessments of how well research systems carry out their essential functions, though one survey of health systems research in 26 countries investigated the type of research being done, the capacity for carrying it out, and the use of research findings in practice (Box 4.2).

To show how to build research systems that can support universal health coverage, this chapter sets out the principles underpinning each of the four key functions, and uses examples to show how they work. The chapter then identifies mechanisms to support these functions, nationally and internationally, through monitoring, coordination and financing. The presentation is intended to be an overview of the research process, not a comprehensive manual. For those who are engaged in building or developing health research systems, whether at provincial, national or regional levels, some of the practical details can be found in a growing number of operational guides, though these

Box 4.1.   WHO's Strategy on Research for Health

In 2010 the Sixty-third World Health Assembly adopted Resolution WHA63.21 concerning a strategy for the management and organization of research within WHO. The World Health Assembly resolution was a stimulus to review and revitalize the role of research within WHO, improve support to WHO Member States in building health research capacity, strengthen advocacy for the importance of research for health, and better communicate WHO's involvement in research for health (1, 2).

Three criteria underpin the WHO approach to health research:

▪ Quality – making a commitment to high-quality research that is ethical, expertly reviewed, efficient, effective, accessible to all, and carefully monitored and evaluated.

▪ Impact – giving priority to research and innovation that has the greatest potential to improve global health security, accelerate health-related development, redress health inequities and attain the MDGs.

▪ Inclusiveness – working in partnership with Member States and stakeholders, taking a multisectoral approach to research for health, and promoting the participation of communities and civil society in the research process.

The strategy has five goals. The first goal applies to WHO while the others apply more generally to the conduct of research (Box 2.1). The goals are:

▪ organization (reinforcing the research culture across WHO);
▪ priorities (emphasizing research that addresses the most important health problems);
▪ capacity (helping to develop and strengthen national health research systems);
▪ standards (promoting good practice in research, setting norms and standards);
▪ translation (linking policy, practice and the products of research).

The global strategy is being used to guide regional and national strategies, taking into account the local context, public health needs and research priorities.

MDGs, Millennium Development Goals.

are not yet comprehensive (4–9). The examples in this chapter, taken together with the body of experience summarized in preceding chapters, lead to some specific recommendations about developing the research environment, especially in low- and middle-income countries.

Setting research priorities

Confronted with an unending list of questions about public health, researchers and policy-makers must together decide which should be given priority for investigation, and thus priority for spending. What follows is a step-by-step guide to setting priorities, highlighting the key questions (1).

▪ Context. What is the exercise about and who is it for? What resources are available?

What are the underlying values or principles? What are the health, research and political environments?

▪ Approach. Should one of the standard approaches be adopted, or do circumstances require the development of new or adjusted methods? Three standard approaches are:
  – 3D Combined Approach Matrix (CAM) – the structured collection of information (10);
  – Essential National Health Research (ENHR) – health research priority-setting for national exercises (11, 12);
  – the Child Health and Nutrition Research Initiative (CHNRI) approach – a systematic algorithm for deciding on priorities (13, 14).

Box 4.2.   A 26-country survey of the status of health systems research

Evaluations of the status of health research are still rare, but one study qualitatively assessed health systems research in 26 low- and middle-income countries in Africa, Asia and South America, as illustrated in the figure (*3*).

Countries surveyed on health systems research

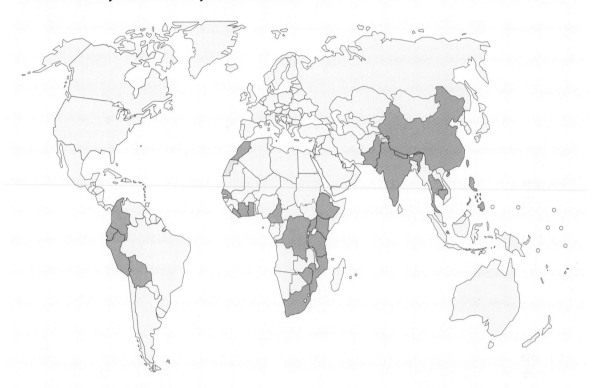

The following conclusions were drawn:

- Low-income countries carried out less health systems research than middle-income countries, but some middle-income countries still had very little research capacity.
- Most African countries have little research capacity, with some exceptions such as Ghana and South Africa. In Asia, India lags behind China.
- Research training programmes are limited or nonexistent in most countries.
- Middle-income countries have greater numbers of researchers and a more diverse disciplinary mix than low-income countries.
- Research in low-income countries tends to be driven by donors, international agencies or international consortia. External funding still plays a big role in many middle-income countries.
- In more than half of the countries surveyed, interest in health systems research has been growing steadily.
- In about two thirds of the countries under evaluation, some evidence-informed decision-making occurs, but not for all health policies.
- A small number of countries showed a preference for the use of domestic evidence or locally-adjusted international best practices (notably China and Thailand).

- Inclusiveness. Who should be involved in setting research priorities and why? Is there an appropriate balance of expertise and interests? Have all relevant parts of the health sector and other constituencies been included? Different constituencies may have their own approaches to setting research priorities (e.g. on health technology assessment or on health policy in the United Kingdom) (*15, 16*).
- Information. What information should be gathered to inform the exercise (e.g. literature reviews, technical data on the burden of disease or on cost–effectiveness, stakeholder views, impact analyses of previous priority-setting exercises)?
- Planning. How will established priorities be turned into research studies? Who will carry out and fund the research?
- Criteria. What factors should determine priorities in any given setting?
- Methods. Should the approach be based on consensus or metrics, or both?
- Evaluation. How will evaluation of the established priorities and the priority-setting process take place? How frequently will such assessments be made?
- Transparency. After the exercise has been completed, what documentation will record how the process was actually carried out, who will prepare it, and how will the findings be made widely known?

These standard methods, which have been expressed in various ways, are steadily being adopted and adapted around the world, and they are producing results that are increasingly transparent and replicable (*17*). However, they have evolved largely from setting research priorities for selected health topics (Box 4.3). So far, attempts to set national priorities for research, across all aspects of health, have not usually been well documented, and there is little

information about whether and how the setting of priorities has influenced the resources allocated to research. Moreover, there has been little emphasis on carrying out cross-disciplinary research, despite agreement on its importance (*42*). The value of cross-disciplinary research has recently been restated by the TB Research Movement (*27, 43*).

The few published national priority-setting exercises that have already been undertaken, such as that in Brazil (Box 4.4), offer lessons for those that will follow (*44–47*). Tomlinson et al. systematically examined how research priorities were set in eight countries, considering the methods used, documentation and legitimacy of the approach, stakeholder involvement, the process of revision and appeals, and leadership (*47*). They found weaknesses in several of the steps outlined above: priorities were typically framed in broad disease categories rather than as specific research questions, engagement with stakeholders was weak, the exercises were poorly documented, and there were no procedures for appealing against the decisions reached. All the exercises were based on internationally-recognized standard methods, but the application of these methods was incomplete.

Strengthening research capacity

Chapter 2 showed how scientific research capacity typically grows disproportionately with national wealth. In the example given, a 10-fold increase in wealth (measured as GNI per capita) has the potential to increase research output (publications or numbers of researchers per capita) by a factor of 50. However, the current research productivity of many countries lies well below this potential (*48*). How then can nations develop the capacity to exploit the full potential of health research?

Box 4.3.   Setting priorities for research on selected health topics

The majority of priority-setting exercises in health research have focused on specific topics. They have typically been carried out from the perspective of different thematic groups within the research community rather than being initiated by national governments. A selection of examples is listed in the table below.

Priority-setting for research on specific topics

Health topic	Focus
Preterm births and stillbirths	Community level (*18*)
Birth asphyxia	Reducing mortality (*19*)
Childhood pneumonia	Reducing mortality (*20*)
Childhood diarrhoea	Reducing mortality (*21*)
Child health	South Africa (*22*)
Mental health	Low- and middle-income countries (*23*)
Mental health and psychosocial support	Humanitarian settings (*24*)
Tuberculosis	From R&D to operational research (*25–28*)
Malaria	Eradication: drugs (*29*)
Malaria	Eradication: health systems and operational research (*30*)
Leishmaniasis	Middle East and North Africa (*31*)
Leishmaniasis	Vaccines (*32*)
Chagas disease, human African trypanosomiasis and leishmaniasis	Diagnostics, drugs, vaccines, vector control and health systems (*33*)
Neglected infectious diseases	Latin America and the Caribbean (*34*)
Helminth infections	Epidemiology and interventions against all major human helminths (*35*)
Zoonoses and infections of marginalized human populations	Epidemiology and interventions; research within and beyond the health sector (*36*)
Noncommunicable diseases	Low- and middle-income countries (*37*)
Human resources for health	Low- and middle-income countries (*38*)
Health systems financing	"Developing" countries (*39*)
Research and development for a national health service	Interface between primary and secondary care in the United Kingdom (*40*)
Equity and health	Social determinants of health (*41*)

R&D, research and development.

A framework for strengthening capacity

The term "capacity" could refer to all elements of a research system. But here it means the abilities of individuals, institutions and networks, nationally and internationally, to undertake and disseminate research findings of the highest quality (*7*). The general principles have been framed by the ESSENCE on Health Research initiative. ESSENCE is a collaboration between funding agencies that aims to improve the impact of investments in institutions and people, and provide enabling mechanisms to address needs and priorities within national strategies on research for health. The principles are as follows (*5*):

- Participation and alignment – a common effort of funders and local partners is

Box 4.4.   Setting priorities for research in Brazil

Since 2000, the Brazilian government has made health research a national priority (*44*). Public resources have been used for fundamental and translational research (see definitions in Box 2.1), and to build closer links between the research community and health services. In 2004, Brazil's National Agenda of Priorities in Health Research was established to help reach the health-related MDGs – i.e. to reduce child mortality, to improve maternal health, and to combat HIV/AIDS, tuberculosis and malaria. The fair allocation of research funds has been guided by six objectives, namely: (i) to improve population health, (ii) to overcome inequity and discrimination, (iii) to respect life and dignity, (iv) to ensure high ethical standards in research, (v) to respect methodological and philosophical plurality, and (vi) to ensure social inclusion, environmental protection and sustainability.

Attempting to satisfy these goals, Brazil's top 10 investments in health research for the period 2004–2009 are shown below.. Most funds were allocated to the "industrial health complex" (biotechnology, equipment and materials, health and technology service providers), to clinical research and to communicable diseases. Among the top 10 investments, but ranked in lower positions, were women's health, mental health and health systems research.

....

Brazil's top ten investments in health research, 2004–2009

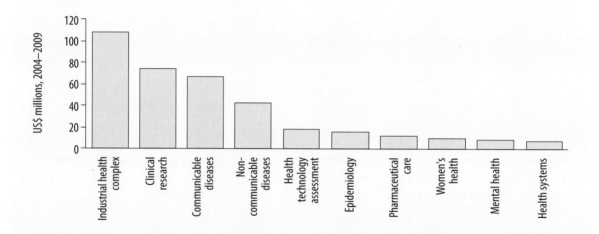

Note: The industrial health complex is described in the text. Health technology assessment includes specific research studies, systematic reviews and economic evaluations.
Source: Pacheco Santos et al.(*44*).

Some 4000 research grants were awarded during this period, and around US$ 545 million were invested in health research across the country by 2010. The south-east region (including Rio de Janeiro and Sao Paulo) carried out 40% of all projects and received 60% of funds. The research has helped to improve treatments, prevention and diagnoses, to develop new products and services, and to strengthen the patient-oriented health-care system (*44*). Priorities are updated periodically, as in the 2011 report *Strategic investigations for the health system*, which identifies 151 research topics based on Brazil's national health policy for 2012–2015.

AIDS, acquired immunodeficiency syndrome; HIV, human immunodeficiency virus; MDGs, Millennium Development Goals.

Box 4.5.   The role of health ministries in developing research capacity: the examples of Guinea Bissau and Paraguay

The **Guinea Bissau** health research system has evolved under the strong influence of international donors and technical partners who have provided funds and scientific expertise (*51*). Research has been carried out chiefly by the Bandim Health Project, the National Laboratory for Public Health, the Department of Epidemiology and the Instituto Nacional de Estudos e Pesquisa (INEP) which is oriented to the social sciences. Research priorities have been set largely by expatriate researchers and have focused on understanding and reducing child mortality.

Recognizing the need to set national research priorities, align funding, build local research capacity and link research to decision-making, the Ministry of Health established the National Institute of Public Health (INASA) in 2010. INASA's role is to coordinate the management and governance of health research nationally. External technical support is led by the West African Health Organisation (WAHO), which works in partnership with the Council on Health Research for Development (COHRED) and the International Development Research Centre (IDRC).

The commitment of the Ministry of Health to invest in research has been central to success. The main challenges facing Guinea Bissau are the limited number of skilled researchers and dependence on foreign assistance.

Paraguay has a stronger research base than Guinea Bissau, with more staff and institutions engaged in health research.[a] However, there has been little coordination between research institutions. In 2007, therefore, the Ministry of Health formed a new directorate for research and in 2009 set up an inter-institutional committee to create a framework for health research. The committee included the Minister of Education and representatives of UNICEF and the Pan American Health Organization. Drawing on the experience of other countries, and especially Mexico, the committee drafted a government policy on research for health and set up the first National Council of Research for Health.

As part of the drive to improve health research, all research institutions in the country are under evaluation. An online database of researchers has been created, and only registered researchers are eligible for funding from the Council of Science and Technology. The database provides information about the training of researchers, their experience, and current research topics. The intention is to manage dedicated funding through a health research trust and to allocate these funds transparently on merit.

As in Guinea Bissau, the support of the Minister of Health backed by the President of Paraguay has been a key factor in the development of a national health research system.

[a] COHRED, personal communication; www.healthresearchweb.org/en/paraguay

needed, with local coordination, in line with the Paris Declaration on Aid Effectiveness (2005), the Accra Agenda for Action (2008), and the broader aim of effective development (*49, 50*).

- Understanding the context – starting with an analysis of the local political, social and cultural norms and practices.
- Building on strengths – local expertise and local processes, initiatives and institutions should be valued rather than bypassed.
- Long-term commitment – there should be recognition that it takes time (years) for inputs to bring about changes in behaviour and performance.

- Interlinked capacity components on different levels – capacity development should take into account the links between individual, organizational and systemic components of health research.
- Continuous learning – this should include an accurate analysis of the situation at the start of the intervention and should allow time to reflect on subsequent action.
- Harmonization – funders, governments and other organizations that support the same partner in capacity-strengthening should harmonize their efforts.

Fig. 4.1.   **Examples of efforts to build research capacity, ranging from individual to global movements**

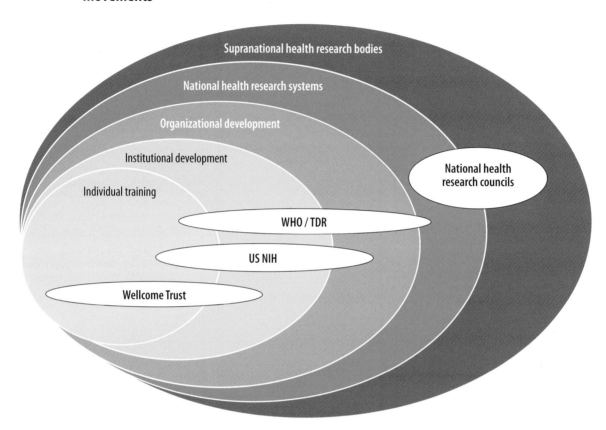

TDR, Special Programme for Research and Training in Tropical Diseases; US NIH, United States National Institutes for Health. Adapted, by permission of the publisher, from Lansang & Dennis (52).

The decision to build and strengthen research capacity, and to allocate the necessary funds, is largely political (Box 4.5), but the case for support must be made with a careful evaluation of what it takes to do research effectively. The needs include a skilled and self-confident workforce with strong leadership, adequate funding with transparent and accountable methods for allocating funds, and well equipped research institutions and networks.

One framework for capacity-building, which has the ingredients of many others, is represented in Fig. 4.1 and Table 4.1 (52–56). While it is useful to begin with structures of this kind, the approach to capacity-building in any setting depends on the strategic vision for the research and what is needed from research. It is sometimes, though not always, convenient to think of institutions nested within organizations. Thus the Task Force on Malaria Research Capability Strengthening in Africa is part of the Multilateral Initiative on Malaria, which is coordinated by the Special Programme for Research and Training in Tropical Diseases (TDR).

Views also differ on the emphasis to be placed on, for example, building elite institutions, creating international networks, boosting translational research, methods of sharing knowledge and information, and rewarding quality (57). Furthermore, there are interactions between the

Table 4.1.   A framework to guide capacity-building, highlighting approaches and targets, the likelihood of sustainability, and the research focus

Entity targeted	Approach to capacity strengthening			
	Graduate or postgraduate training	Learning by doing	Institutional partnerships between countries	Centres of excellence
Individual[a]	+++	+	++	+
Institution	+++	++	+++	+++
Network	++	++	+++	++
National level	+	++	++	+++
Supranational level		++	+++	++
Financial investment[b]	++	+	+++	+++
Research focus	Research skills	→		Programme, policy, systems development
Likelihood of sustainability[c]	+	→		+++

[a] Plus (+) signs indicate the entity is targeted + sometimes, ++ often, +++ frequently.

[b] Plus (+) signs in this row indicate that the extent of financial investment needed by national health research systems or funding agencies is + low, ++ medium, +++ high.

[c] Plus signs in this row indicate the likelihood of sustainability of various approaches is + fair, +++ strong.

Reproduced, by permission of the publisher, from Lansang & Dennis (52).

various components in Table 4.1. For instance, graduate and postgraduate training are more likely to be effective when the host institutions are also strong (Table 4.1, column 1, row 2).

From the outset, any programme to strengthen research capacity must define, monitor and evaluate success – an area in which knowledge is still sparse (52, 53, 58–60). A simple geographical mapping of research activity can be illuminating (Fig. 4.2), but a deeper understanding comes from measuring success. One evaluation examined which indicators of research capacity were most useful in four different settings: evidence-based health care in Ghana, HIV voluntary counselling and testing services in Kenya, poverty as a determinant of access to TB services in Malawi, and the promotion of community health in the Democratic Republic of the Congo (6). The most expedient indicators changed as programmes matured. The engagement of stakeholders and planning for scale-up were critical at the outset, while innovation, financial resources, and the institutionalization

of activities mattered more during the expansion stage. Funding for core activities and local management were vital during the consolidation stage.

The following sections look more closely at three elements of capacity that are universally important: building the research workforce, tracking financial flows, and developing institutions and networks.

Creating and retaining a skilled research workforce

The world health report 2006 – working together for health highlighted the critical role, and the chronic shortage, of health workers, especially in low-income countries (62). Here the vital contribution made by health researchers as part of the health workforce is underscored (56, 63).

The research carried out in many low- and middle-income countries is still dominated by scientists from wealthier countries who bring

Fig. 4.2. **Geographical distribution of research capacity in Africa**

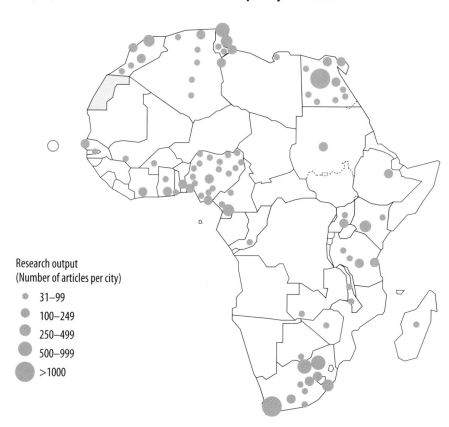

Research output
(Number of articles per city)
- 31–99
- 100–249
- 250–499
- 500–999
- >1000

R&D, research and development.
Note: Mapping of top 40 African cities by research output shows hotspots and coldspots of R&D activity and highlights inequities in R&D productivity across the continent.
Adapted with the World Health Organization's map shapefile under the Creative Commons licence (CC BY 3.0, http://creativecommons.org/licenses/by/3.0/) from Nwaka et al. (*61*).

much-needed expertise and funding. The transition towards a more self-reliant and skilled research workforce in lower-income countries is under way, but the process is slow.

International collaboration is part of the solution so long as some basic principles are followed (Box 4.6). Alongside the numerous examples of "north–south" research collaboration run a variety of training schemes for young researchers – such as those offered by TDR (www.who.int/tdr), the Training Programs in Epidemiology and Public Health Interventions Network

(TEPHINET), www.tephinet.org), the European Foundation Initiative for African Research into Neglected Tropical Diseases (EFINTD, www.ntd-africa.net), Brazil's Science without Borders programme (www.cienciasemfronteiras.gov.br), and the product-orientated operational research courses offered by the International Union against Tuberculosis and Lung Disease and Médecins Sans Frontières (MSF) Luxembourg (*65–67*). Even where there are shortages of money to do the research in Africa, there is an appetite for career development through mentorship

Box 4.6.   **Principles of research partnership**

Further details of these 11 principles can be found in *Guidelines for research in partnership with developing countries* prepared by the Swiss Commission for Research Partnership with Developing Countries (*64*). The 11 principles (with minor adaptation) are as follows:

1. Decide on research objectives together, including those who will use the results.

2. Build mutual trust, stimulating honest and open research collaboration.

3. Share information and develop networks for coordination.

4. Share responsibility and ownership.

5. Create transparency in financial and other transactions.

6. Monitor and evaluate collaboration, judging performance through regular internal and 1. external evaluations.

7. Disseminate the results through joint publications and other means, with adequate communication to those who will finally use them.

8. Apply the results as far as is possible, recognizing the obligation to ensure that results are used to benefit the target group.

9. Share the benefits of research profits equitably including any profit, publications and patents.

10. Increase research capacity at individual and institutional levels.

11. Build on the achievements of research – especially new knowledge, sustainable development and research capacity.

programmes, project management courses, proposal-writing workshops and language training, and by networking at conferences (*65*).

Through these various schemes, scientists in lower-income countries are gaining a more confident voice. For instance, African researchers have argued that support for research on neglected tropical diseases should not be the sole responsibility of external donors. They believe that their own governments must also take responsibility for providing infrastructure and job opportunities (*65, 68*).

Ensuring transparency and accountability in research funding

Just as research needs money, the development of research capacity needs a mechanism for tracking how much is spent on what kinds of research. The eight areas of research outlined in Box 2.2 – ranging from fundamental or underpinning studies to investigations of health systems and services – offer one framework for reporting

the money spent on research in different areas. In the United Kingdom, for instance, research spending by the Wellcome Trust and Medical Research Council (MRC) focuses on underpinning and etiological research (Fig. 4.3). In contrast, research spending by two national health departments (England and Scotland) is oriented to treatment evaluation, disease management and health services (*69, 70*). These are different but complementary and point to funding gaps that need to be filled, perhaps from other sources. The data in Fig. 4.3 indicate that the Wellcome Trust, the MRC and the health departments provide relatively little money for research on prevention (group 3) or on detection and diagnosis (group 4). This is an argument not only for research monitoring but also for greater harmonization between funding bodies.

The virtues of having a standard method of accounting for research funds are clear – for communication, comparability and collaboration (*69*). The approach illustrated in Fig. 4.3 is one scheme among a number that have been

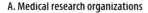

Fig. 4.3. **Contrasting but complementary profiles of health research spending, United Kingdom of Great Britain and Northern Ireland, 2009–2010**

A. Medical research organizations

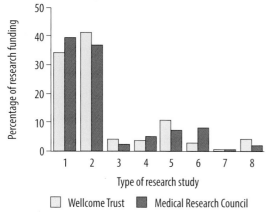

B. National health departments

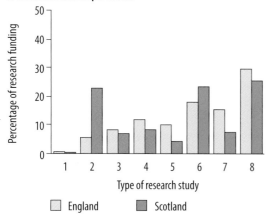

Types of research: 1, underpinning; 2, etiology; 3, prevention; 4, detection and diagnosis; 5, treatment development; 6, treatment evaluation; 7, disease management; 8, health systems and services (Box 2.2).

Note: For each of the four organizations, percentages sum to 100%.

Adapted, by permission of the publisher, from the UK Clinical Research Collaboration (69).

proposed (69). All take a similar approach to classification – a disease code is combined with a description of the research purpose – indicating that there is a common understanding of what a classification system should include. The next step in reconciling different schemes could take one of two directions: either agreement to adopt the same system, or reliance on computer software to translate and map the current variety of classification systems to a common standard (71). The best approach will be the one that most easily achieves the main goal, which is to assure transparency and accountability in research funding (70).

The amount of funding sought for research should be based on an assessment of what studies are needed and how much they cost. Despite the importance of good accounting in research, the evaluation of both need and cost are underdeveloped skills.

Funding for TB operational research illustrates the challenge of assessing need. The desirable expenditure (budget) for TB operational research has been set at US$ 80 million annually, calculated as 1% of the expenditure of national TB control programmes (72). Against this arbitrary spending target, which is far lower than that for any other area of TB research, the available funds totalled 76% of assessed need. This is a higher percentage than for any other area of research (Fig. 4.4) (73). The danger here is to conclude that the need for operational research has largely been satisfied. While the Global Plan to Stop TB has successfully highlighted the need to invest in R&D for technology, a more objective method is needed for calculating the TB operational research budget, especially in light of the widely-held view that too little effort is devoted to operational research (28, 74, 75).

On the question of costing, the calculation of direct expenditure is relatively straightforward. It refers to the indirect costs that are harder to define, including the funds needed to build and upgrade infrastructure (76). Research institutions

Fig. 4.4.   Global expenditures and budget gap in tuberculosis R&D by research category, 2010

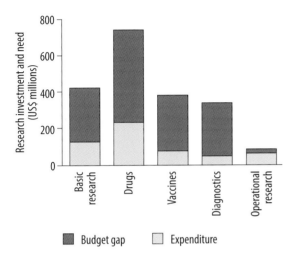

R&D, research and development.
Note: Relatively little money is spent on diagnostics and operational research; the budget for operational research is exceptionally low.
Reproduced, by permission of the publisher, from Treatment Action Group (73).

in low- and middle-income countries have the task of persuading external donors to contribute to indirect costs, and also to align their research priorities in contributing to direct costs. Both of these problems were confronted – and solved – by the International Centre for Diarrhoeal Diseases Research, Bangladesh (ICDDR,B) in 2006 (77). Solutions were found, in part by adopting a transparent approach to financial monitoring and evaluation. ICDDR,B explicitly defined and measured activities, outputs and outcomes in the areas of research, clinical services, teaching, and management and operations.

Building research institutions and networks

The Global Health Trials network has expressed a view of capacity-building that is shared by other health research networks (Box 4.7). In the context of research networks, "capacity" is seen as the establishment of a community of researchers based in lower-income countries who can devise and validate methods and operational tools for improving health, and who share local and global solutions to make pragmatic and locally-led development possible (79). Box 4.8 describes the success of a multinational network that successfully evaluated the diagnosis and treatment of syphilis.

Putting the spotlight on collaboration between lower-income countries does not mean neglecting the traditional links through which higher-income countries continue to provide funds and expertise to those with lower incomes and where the emphasis of the research studies of each group differs from that of the other group but both are complementary. For instance, clinical trials in poorer countries have focused largely on communicable rather than noncommunicable diseases. In contrast, researchers in richer countries have enormous expertise in studying noncommunicable diseases. Their expertise will be in demand as the need for research on these diseases continues to rise worldwide (79).

Defining and implementing norms and standards

Codes of practice for the responsible conduct of research have been written by many research organizations around the world. Among them are the United Kingdom's Medical Research Council

Box 4.7.   Developing research networks

Initiative to Strengthen Health Research Capacity in Africa (ISHReCA)

ISHReCA (ishreca.org) is an African-led initiative whose mission is to build strong foundations for health research in Africa (*55, 59*). ISHReCA aims to expand research capacity in four ways: (i) it provides a platform for African health researchers to discuss ways of building sustainable capacity for health research in Africa; (ii) it promotes an African-led agenda for health research, negotiating with funders and partners concerning support for, and harmonization of, research initiatives; (iii) it advocates for increased commitment to research by national governments and civil society, emphasizing the translation of research into policy and practice; and (iv) it seeks novel ways to garner regional and international support for health research in Africa.

African Network for Drugs and Diagnostics Innovation (ANDI)

Launched in 2008, ANDI (www.andi-africa.org) is hosted by the United Nations Economic Commission for Africa (UNECA) in Addis Ababa (*61*). Backed by the first African-owned and managed innovation fund, ANDI's mission is to "promote and sustain African-led health product innovation to address African public health needs through efficient use of local knowledge, assembly of research networks, and building of capacity to support economic development". The vision is to create a sustainable platform for R&D innovation that addresses Africa's own health needs. To realize this vision, ANDI is building capacity that supports pharmaceutical research, development and manufacturing to improve access to medicines. Specific activities include the development of a portfolio of high-quality, pan-African pharmaceutical R&D innovation projects, project coordination and management, including intellectual property management. Vital to ANDI are more than 30 African institutions which are recognized as research centres of excellence and are committed to sharing expertise, knowledge, research equipment and facilities (*61, 78*).

Global Health Trials

Global Health Trials (globalhealthtrials.tghn.org) is an online community that shares information on clinical studies and experimental trials in global health, providing guidance, tools, resources, training and professional development. An e-learning centre offers short courses, seminars and a library.

Pan-African Consortium for the Evaluation of Anti-Tuberculosis Antibiotics (PanACEA)

North–south research collaboration, such as that fostered by the **European and Developing Countries Clinical Trials Partnership** (www.edctp.org), has existed for many years. The EDCTP 14-country partnership works to "accelerate the development of new or improved drugs, vaccines, microbicides and diagnostics against HIV/AIDS, tuberculosis and malaria, with a focus on phase II and III clinical trials in sub-Saharan Africa".

An offshoot of EDCTP, PanACEA is a network of 11 linked clinical trial sites in six African countries, supported by European research organizations and pharmaceutical companies. The initial aim of the network was to investigate the role of moxifloxacin in reducing treatment durations for TB. However, PanACEA has a wider ambition – to establish collaboration rather than competition as a driving force in the conduct of high-quality clinical and regulatory trials.

Research for Health Africa (R4HA)

The goal of R4HA (www.cohred.org/r4ha) is to solve common problems through collective action. The NEPAD Agency and COHRED, financially supported by the Ministry of Foreign Affairs of the Netherlands, work with Mozambique, Senegal and Tanzania to strengthen the governance of research for health in these countries. Country focused activities are complemented by cross-country learning and exchange opportunities. At the same time, in 2011, a group of 14 West African countries launched a four-year project dedicated to strengthening health research systems. The project is financed by Canada's IDRC and the West African Health Organisation (WAHO), with technical facilitation provided by COHRED. An assessment of research for health in this group of West African countries identified Guinea-Bissau, Liberia, Mali and Sierra Leone as most in need of support. WAHO and COHRED help to build the research systems in these countries based on action plans they have defined themselves.

R&D, research and development.

Box 4.8.   How to prevent and treat syphilis: an operational research network connecting six countries

Two million pregnant women are infected with syphilis each year. More than half transmit the infection to newborn children, resulting in premature births, stillbirths and underweight babies. Syphilis also augments sexual and mother-to-child transmission of HIV.

However, syphilis is easily diagnosed and treated, and congenital syphilis is preventable. Point-of-care diagnostic tests and treatment with penicillin each cost less than US$ 1. The London School of Hygiene & Tropical Medicine coordinated a three-year, multicountry implementation research project to determine the feasibility and cost–effectiveness of using simple diagnostic tests and same-day treatment in prenatal and high-risk populations in low- and middle-income countries (*80*). More than 150 000 individuals were screened in six countries. Interventions were introduced through existing services, so there was no need for new infrastructure.

Numbers screened and population focus by country

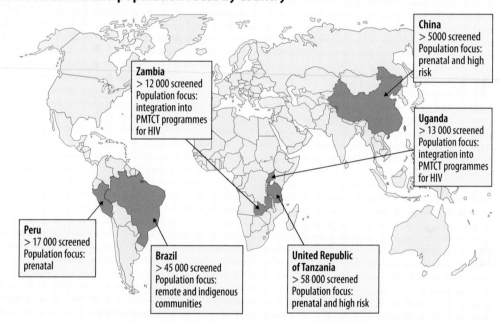

Initial preparatory work – including making sure that screening was culturally acceptable – was critical to the success of the project. In China, female sex workers were trained to speak to other female sex workers and encourage them to take up screening. In a seventh country, Haiti, traditional healers were educated about the signs and symptoms of syphilis, which enabled them to refer patients to health clinics.

Ministries of health were consulted about what evidence they would need before considering a change of policy. A baseline survey of services and barriers aided the design of specific interventions to overcome obstacles and to measure increase in coverage. Health ministries were given regular updates which provided a sense of ownership and facilitated policy change. From staffing to equipment, emphasis was placed on establishing systems that could be sustained.

In all participating countries, the study achieved significant increases in coverage of diagnostic testing for syphilis. This reduced the prevalence of syphilis and the risk of HIV infection. Some benefits were immediately visible and led to rapid policy changes which were, in some instances, implemented even before the research studies were completed.

The research also helped to strengthen health services in some of the participating countries. In Brazil, for instance, it has provided a model for the provision of health services to indigenous populations, as well as a template for the introduction of new technologies.

PMTCT, Prevention of mother-to-child transmission.

and Australia's National Health and Medical Research Council (*81, 82*). This section outlines the main responsibilities that fall on institutions and researchers in carrying out responsible research. Because these principles are laid out clearly in international guidelines, the task is not necessarily to develop the principles further but to see that they are applied everywhere.

Ethics and ethical review

The ethical principles that guide the behaviour of researchers, overseen by ethical committees, are to ensure honesty, objectivity, integrity, justice, accountability, intellectual property, professional courtesy and fairness, the protection of participants in research studies, and good stewardship of research on behalf of others (*83–88*).

WHO has defined 10 standards that should be met in ethical reviews of health research with human participants (Box 4.9). These standards are designed to complement existing laws, regulations and practices, and to serve as a basis on which research ethics committees can develop their own specific practices and written procedures. Among the organizations that monitor compliance with ethical standards are independent bodies such as the United Kingdom's Research Integrity Office (www.ukrio.org) and the Wemos Foundation (www.wemos.nl).

Reporting and sharing research data, tools and materials

The research community is responsible for ensuring the accuracy of methods, integrity of results, production and sharing of data, adequacy of peer review, and protection of intellectual property (*81, 90, 91*).

In the era of open access, an influential body of opinion synthesized by the United Kingdom's Royal Society holds that "intelligent openness" should become the norm in scientific research (*92*). This means openness of researchers with other scientists and with the public and media;

greater recognition of the value of data-gathering, analysis and communication; common standards for sharing information; mandatory publication of data in a reusable form to support findings; and the development of expertise and software for managing the enormous volume of digital data (*93*). In this Royal Society review, intelligent openness is seen as the key to scientific progress. It is the basis for understanding and communicating results that can be exploited for practical purposes, including the improvement of health.

Accompanying this general trend towards openness is a proliferation of Internet-based platforms for sharing information. Among these are the Health Research Web, Health Systems Evidence, and PDQ-Evidence (Box 4.10). As data exchange becomes commonplace, consistent database structures and standards for reporting are needed for efficient communication. The principles and practice for sharing genomic data are well advanced but those for sharing data on innovation, research and development are less developed (*94, 95*).

Registering clinical trials

The Declaration of Helsinki (1964–2008) states that "every clinical trial must be registered in a publicly accessible database before recruitment of the first subject". The registration of clinical trials is a scientific, ethical and moral responsibility because decisions about health care must be informed by all of the available evidence. From a practical standpoint, the International Clinical Trials Registry Platform (ICTRP) helps researchers and funding agencies to avoid unnecessary duplication, to identify gaps in clinical trials research, and to find out about trials in which they may have an interest and with which they might collaborate (*96*). In addition, the process of registration has the potential to improve the quality of clinical trials – e.g. by revealing problems in design at an early stage. Although the regulatory, legal, ethical and funding requirements for the oversight and conduct of clinical

Box 4.9.   **Standards for the ethical review of research with human participants**

These standards (which are abbreviated here) are intended as guidance for research ethics committees and for the researchers who design and carry out health research studies (*88*). The task of ethical review involves more than standing committees and includes, for example, independent teams of trained external assessors that can investigate allegations of research misconduct (*89*).

1. Responsibility for establishing the research ethics review system

Ethical review must be supported by an adequate legal framework. Research ethics committees must be able to provide independent reviews of all health-related research at national, subnational and/or institutional (public or private) levels.

2. Composition of research ethics committees

Research ethics committees should have multidisciplinary and multisectoral membership, including individuals with relevant research expertise.

3. Research ethics committee resources

Research ethics committees should have adequate resources – staff, facilities and finance – to carry out their responsibilities.

4. Independence of research ethics committees

The independence of research ethics committee operations must be ensured in order to protect decision-making from influence by any individual or entity that sponsors, conducts or hosts the research it reviews.

5. Training the research ethics committee

Training should be provided on the ethical aspects of health-related research with human participants, on the application of ethical considerations to different types of research, and on the conduct of research reviews by the research ethics committee.

6. Transparency, accountability and quality of the research ethics committee

Mechanisms exist to make the operations of research ethics committees transparent, accountable, consistent and of high quality.

7. The ethical basis for decision-making in research ethics committees

The research ethics committee bases its decisions about the research that it reviews on a coherent and consistent application of the ethical principles that are articulated in international guidance documents and human rights instruments, as well as on any national laws or policies consistent with those principles.

8. Decision-making procedures for research ethics committees

Decisions on research protocols are based on a thorough and inclusive process of discussion and deliberation.

9. Written policies and procedures

Written policies and procedures include specification of the membership of the research ethics committee, committee governance, review procedures, decision-making, communications, follow-up and monitoring, documentation and archiving, training, quality assurance, and procedures for coordination with other research ethics committees.

10. Researchers' responsibilities

Research is performed only by persons with scientific, clinical or other relevant qualifications appropriate to the project, who carry out the research in compliance with the requirements established by the research ethics committee.

Box 4.10. Sharing information on current practice in health research: some examples

Health Research Web (www.healthresearchweb.org) provides data, tables and graphs for monitoring and evaluating research investments at national or institutional level. The platform uses an editable wiki-type format so that institutions and agencies can personalize entries to suit their own needs. The information presented includes research policies, priorities, projects, capacities and outputs, as illustrated in the following figure.

The Health Research Web

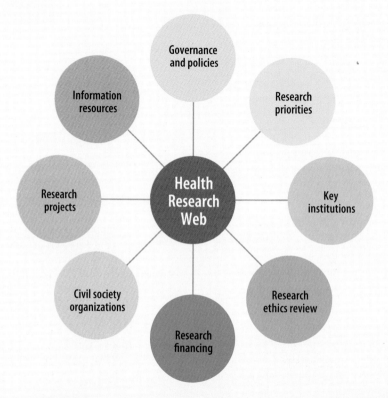

The number of users of the platform is growing at both regional and country levels. In the Americas, the Pan American Health Organization (PAHO) has developed Health Research Web – Americas (www.healthresearchweb. org/en/americas), which is linked to EVIPNet (Box 4.12) and to hundreds of research ethics committees active in Latin America. In Africa, the Tanzanian Commission for Science and Technology (COSTECH) uses the platform to issue public calls for research proposals. With this platform COSTECH can monitor which studies have been supported, see how these respond to national research priorities, check what public resources are allocated to the research, and consult the research findings.

Health Systems Evidence (www.healthsystemsevidence.org), an initiative of the McMaster Health Forum, is a continuously updated repository of evidence – mainly systematic reviews – about the governance and financing of health systems and the delivery of health services.

PDQ-Evidence (www.pdq-evidence.org), maintained by the Evidence-Based Medicine unit of the Pontificia Universidad Católica de Chile (Pontifical Catholic University of Chile), also provides evidence about public health and about health systems and services. Information is presented mainly in the form of structured summaries and systematic reviews.

trials differ between countries, the ICTRP is a worldwide resource that can be used for clinical trials wherever they are carried out. Since 2000, the number of registered clinical trials has increased markedly, and there are now more than 200 000 records on the ICTRP.

Using evidence to develop policy, practice and products

Good practice dictates that any findings that might have an impact on clinical practice, on the development of methods of prevention or treatment, or on public policy should be made available to those who wish to use them (*81*). However, conveying information is just one part of the process of translating research evidence into health policy and practice, as described in the next section.

Translating evidence into policy and practice

There is a broad consensus that most health research is devoted to developing new interventions and demonstrating their efficacy in experimental trials, and that far too little effort is given to the process of turning evidence from research into actions that improve health (*97, 98*). In the context of achieving universal health coverage, a large number of cheap, efficacious and cost-effective existing interventions remain inaccessible to many who could benefit from them (*99–101*). Some proven interventions are hardly used at all; for others, widespread implementation may take years or decades (Fig. 4.5) (*102*).

A variety of conceptual approaches have been used to map the path from evidence to action – the "triangle that moves the mountain" and others (*103–106*). Notwithstanding the theory, however, the evidence on how rapidly to achieve high coverage of interventions is generally weak (*59, 107*). To simplify the problem by division, four questions help to understand the

Fig. 4.5.   Proportion of 40 low-income countries implementing five interventions, over periods of up to 27 years since regulatory approval

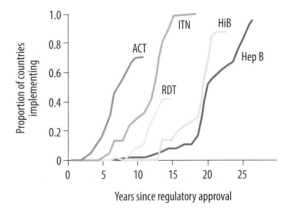

The interventions: ACT, artemisin-based combination therapies; Hep B, Hepatitis B vaccine; HiB, haemophilus influenza type b vaccine; ITN, insecticide-treated mosquito net; RDT, rapid malaria diagnostic test.
Adapted under the Open Access licence from Brooks et al. (*102*).

reasons why interventions of known efficacy are not taken to scale (*108*).

First, how can the results of research be presented in a form that is comprehensible and credible to the population of potential users?

Second, how best can the results, once clearly described, be actively disseminated? In this context, who is the audience and through what channels can they be reached? Box 4.11 contains a checklist of the pitfalls in dissemination, with some guidance on how to avoid them (*111*). Not everyone will agree with all of the remedies. Thus, rather than guarding against premature publicity, Brooks et al. argue that dissemination, which make take decades (Fig. 4.5), can be achieved more quickly by anticipating and removing likely bottlenecks during the R&D phase (*102*).

Box 4.11.   Ten common mistakes in the dissemination of new interventions, and suggestions for avoiding them

1. Assuming that evidence matters to potential adopters

Suggestion: Evidence is most important only to a subset of potential adopters, and is often used to reject proposed interventions. Therefore, emphasize other variables such as compatibility, cost and simplicity when communicating about innovations.

2. Substituting the perceptions of researchers for those of potential adopters

Suggestion: Listen to representatives of the potential adopters to understand their needs and reactions to new interventions.

3. Using intervention creators as intervention communicators

Suggestion: Enable access to experts, but rely on communicators who will elicit the attention of potential adopters.

4. Introducing interventions before they are ready

Suggestion: Publicize interventions only after clear results have been obtained.

5. Assuming that information will influence decision-making

Suggestion: Information is necessary, but influence is usually needed too. Therefore pair sources of information with sources of social and political influence.

6. Confusing authority with influence

Suggestion: Gather data on who among potential adopters is seen as a source of advice and use them to accelerate dissemination.

7. Allowing those who are first to adopt (innovators) to gain primacy in dissemination efforts

Suggestion: Initial adopters are not always typical or influential. Find out how potential adopters and key users are related to each other in order to identify those who are most influential (*109*).

8. Failing to distinguish between change agents, authority figures, opinion leaders and innovation champions

Suggestion: Single individuals do not usually play multiple roles, so determine what part each person can play in the dissemination process.

9. Selecting demonstration sites on criteria of motivation and capacity

Suggestion: The spread of an intervention depends on how initial demonstration sites are seen by others. So, when selecting demonstration sites, consider which sites will have a positive influence.

10. Advocating single interventions as the solution to a problem

Suggestion: One intervention is unlikely to fit all circumstances; offering a cluster of evidence-based practices is usually more effective (*105, 110*).

Adapted from Dearing (*111*).

Third, by what criteria do potential users decide to adopt a new intervention? Ideally, the decision formally to adopt will ultimately be embodied in government policy.

And fourth, once the decision to adopt has been taken, how should an intervention be implemented and evaluated? In practice, there is a tension between preserving the intervention in its original form and adapting it to local circumstances. By and large, programmes can be expected to work imperfectly at first and will need to be adapted and refined (*105*).

To help answer these four questions for a variety of interventions in different settings, an assortment of networks, tools and instruments is available, including EvipNet, SURE, TRAction and SUPPORT (Box 4.12). In the context of health systems performance, the methods for judging

Box 4.12.   Translating research into policy and practice

There is an important distinction between evidence used to set policy and evidence used to influence practice. The first two examples below focus on policy, the third on practice.

Evidence-Informed Policy Networks (EVIPNet)

The purpose of EVIPNet (www.evipnet.org) is to strengthen health systems by linking the results of scientific research to the development of health policy. EVIPNet is a network of teams in more than 20 countries around the world, which synthesize research findings, produce policy briefs, and organize policy forums that bring together policy-makers, researchers and citizen groups. Recent initiatives have, for example, helped to improve access to ACT for the treatment of malaria in Africa and debated the role of primary health care in the management of chronic noncommunicable diseases in the Americas (*112*). As a component of EVIPnet, SURE (Support for the Use of Research Evidence) offers a set of guides for preparing and using policy briefs to support health systems development in Africa.

SUPPORT tools for evidence-informed health policy-making

SUPPORT is a collection of articles that describe how to use scientific evidence to inform health policy (*113*). The series shows, among other things, how to make best use of systematic reviews and how in general to use research evidence to clarify problems linked to health policy.

The Translating Research into Action (TRAction) project

Recognizing that many health problems in developing countries already have solutions that have not been applied, **TRAction** (www.tractionproject.org) promotes wider use of interventions that are known to be effective, awarding grants for translational research in the areas of maternal, newborn and child health. TRAction is part of the Health Research Program (HaRP) of the United States Agency for International Development (USAID).

ACT, artemisin-based combination therapies.

evidence on the effectiveness of interventions are well developed. However, new tools are needed to help assess evidence from systematic reviews in terms of the acceptability of policy options to stakeholders and the feasibility of implementation, and in terms of equity. Research is also needed on ways to develop, structure and present policy options in relation to the functions of health systems (*114, 115*).

Researchers and decision-makers typically work in different communities, and the research described in technical publications and scientific journals cannot easily be evaluated by most of the people who make most of the decisions (see Box 2.3 on the GRADE system for judging evidence for policy and practice) (*116*). The influence of research depends on how research activities are positioned with respect to the bodies that are responsible for setting policy and practice. For maximum effect, health research should be embedded as a core function

in every health system (*54*). A research department located within a health ministry should be well positioned to transfer research findings to policy-makers and to help oversee national research practice – for instance by setting up national databases of research projects approved and completed, of scientific publications produced, and of patents awarded.

When researchers are put in close contact with policy-makers they will be in a position not simply to produce results on demand but also to shape the research agenda (*117*). For instance, routine evaluation of public health programmes is an important source of questions for research, and yet few countries have laws and policies that require such evaluations to be done (*118*). One weakness of existing schemes for promoting universal health coverage is that they fail to involve evaluators from the start (*119*). Research scientists placed in public health programmes would stimulate monitoring and evaluation.

Monitoring and coordinating research, nationally and internationally

Mechanisms to stimulate and facilitate research for universal health coverage include monitoring, coordination and financing. These are closely related and have repeatedly been proposed as ways of promoting and supporting high-priority research (*120–122*). Most recently, the report of the Consultative Expert Working Group on Research and Development: Financing and Coordination (CEWG) made a series of recommendations to support R&D for health technology, and the Alliance on Health Policy and Systems Research did the same for HPSR (Box 4.13) (*117, 123, 124*). Many of the ideas for promoting R&D and HPSR apply to all aspects of health research, so these are drawn together here.

Where there is a commitment to share data, a global observatory, built on national observatories and regional hubs, can in principle do the following in support of research for universal health coverage:

- compile, analyse and present data on financial flows for health;
- act as a repository of data on research findings and on the efficacy, safety, quality and affordability of interventions, including the registration of clinical trials;
- in collaboration with other organizations that currently gather data on science and technology indicators (e.g. UNESCO, OECD, the Network for Science and Technology Indicators – Ibero-American and Inter-American, the World Intellectual Property Organization), bring together information on research publications, clinical trials and patents, as envisaged in the Global Strategy and Plan of Action on Public Health, Innovation and Intellectual Property (Box 2.7) (*125*);
- chart progress on research for universal health coverage by measuring inputs and health impact along the results chain (Chapter 1);

Box 4.13. WHO Strategy on Health Policy and Systems Research

The WHO Strategy on Health Policy and Systems Research (HPSR), launched in November 2012, was shaped by the Alliance on Health Policy and Systems Research. The strategy explains how the evolving field of health policy and systems research (Box 2.1) responds to the information needs of decision-makers, health practitioners and civil society, all of whom are responsible for the planning and performance of national health systems (*117*). As the first-ever global strategy in this area, it represents a milestone in the evolution of HPSR.

The strategy has three aims. First, it seeks to unify the worlds of research and decision-making and connect the various research disciplines that generate knowledge on health systems. Second, it contributes to a broader understanding of the field by clarifying the scope and role of HPSR and providing insights into the dynamic processes through which HPSR evidence is generated and used in decision-making. Third, the strategy is intended to serve as an agent for change, advocating close collaboration between researchers and decision-makers as an alternative to working in parallel.

The strategy document outlines several actions by which stakeholders can facilitate evidence-informed decision-making and strengthen health systems. Some of these actions are reflected in the main text of this chapter. These mutually complementary options support the embedding of research into decision-making processes and promote national and global investment in HPSR. National governments may choose to pursue some or all of these actions on the basis of their individual needs and available resources.

- generate and promote research standards, increase accountability for action, and provide technical support;
- facilitate collaboration and coordination, especially between countries, by sharing information from the repository of data.

Whether all these functions can be satisfied in practice depends on the resources available and the will to develop national, regional and global observatories. These ideas form part of the continuing debate about how to promote R&D for health in low-income countries (126).

Monitoring provides opportunities to coordinate research activities: information-sharing, network-building and collaboration are essential ingredients of coordination. The advantages of coordination lie in jointly developing solutions to common problems, sometimes with shared resources. However, there are disadvantages too. One dilemma in coordination is how to provide opportunities to make research more effective – for instance by seeking to be complementary and to avoid duplication – without imposing undue constraints on creativity and innovation.

At its least complicated, coordination is facilitated simply by sharing information. The observatory Orphanet, for example, is a reference portal that provides information on rare diseases and orphan drugs (127). On a different level, coordination might entail the joint setting of priorities for research on a selected theme, such as interventions to control noncommunicable diseases (37). At a yet higher level of organization, there might be joint research projects, for example to test new tools for prevention or treatment at sites in several countries. Examples are the coordinated evaluation of MenAfriVac across west and central Africa, and the diagnosis and treatment of syphilis on three continents (Box 4.8) (80, 128, 129).

Financing research for universal health coverage

Health research is more productive when there is a guaranteed, regular income. International donors and national governments can measure their own commitments to investing in health research against defined, voluntary benchmarks. A series of benchmarks for research funding has been proposed, and these may be taken as starting points in setting targets for research funding (121). Accordingly, the 1990 Commission on Health Research for Development suggested that each nation should spend at least 2% of national health expenditure on "essential national health research" (120). A more recent recommendation is that "developing" countries should commit 0.05–0.1% of GDP to government-funded health research of all kinds (121). Higher-income countries should commit 0.15–0.2% of GDP to government-funded health research (121). The choice of benchmarks is discretionary but should be commensurate with achieving, or at least lie on a trajectory to, universal health coverage.

National and international governance of health research

One may ask whether the health research system in any country is effectively governed and managed – i.e. whether all the essential functions are carried out to a high standard. Systematic evaluations of research governance are valuable but rare. In one of the few examples, eight indicators of governance and management were used to assess the national health research systems of 10 countries in the WHO Eastern Mediterranean Region (Fig. 4.6) (130).

This evaluation found some examples of good practice, but few countries had a formal national health research system and many of the

Fig. 4.6. **Eight aspects of governance and management of the national health research systems (NHRS) in 10 countries of the Eastern Mediterranean region**

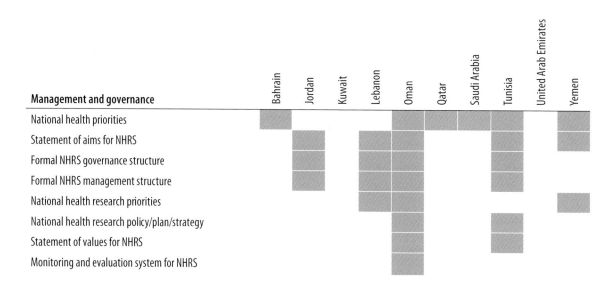

Source: Kennedy et al. (*130*).

basic building blocks of an effective system were not in place. On the basis of these indicators, it was clear that the 10 countries differed greatly in their research capabilities and that the best performers among them were Lebanon, Oman and Tunisia. Similar evaluations have been carried out for Latin American countries and for Pacific island nations (*45, 131*). The best kind of governance ensures that all key functions of a research system are carried out within a regulatory framework that is light enough to facilitate rather than hinder the research process (*132*).

Conclusions: building effective research systems

The four functions of an effective research system – setting priorities, building capacity, setting standards, and translating evidence into practice – are in various stages of development in nations around the world. Consequently, the parts of the system that need most attention vary from one country to another. The conclusion of this overview therefore highlights one aspect of each function that is important for all national health research systems.

First, on choosing topics for research, more effort is needed to set national health research priorities, as distinct from setting priorities for selected health topics.

Second, the capacity of any country to carry out the necessary research depends on funding, institutions and networks. However, it is the people who do research – with their curiosity, imagination, motivation, technical skills, experience and connections – who are most critical to the success of the research enterprise.

Third, codes of practice, which are the cornerstone of any research system, are already in use in many countries. However, they need to be further developed and adapted to new settings and new circumstances. An important task ahead is to ensure adherence to nationally and internationally agreed standards in the conduct of research.

Fourth, although a wide range of fundamental and applied research studies is essential in order to reach universal health coverage, there is a particular need to close the gap between existing knowledge and action. To help close this gap, research should be strengthened, not only in academic centres, but also in public health programmes close to the supply of and demand for health services.

Apart from considering how research is done, especially within countries, this chapter has also outlined methods for supporting research, nationally and internationally. The support is provided by three mechanisms: monitoring, coordination and financing. One way to monitor research more effectively is by establishing linked national and international research observatories. A function of observatories is to aid coordination, through information-sharing and by facilitating collaborative research studies. Observatories can also monitor financial flows for research and can help ensure that there is adequate funding to support research on global and national priorities.

In view of what has already been achieved in research, the next task is to identify what actions can be taken to build more effective research systems. Chapter 5 proposes a set of actions based on the main themes of this report. ■

References

1. Viergever RF et al. A checklist for health research priority setting: nine common themes of good practice. *Health Research Policy and Systems*, 2010,8:36. PMID:21159163.
2. Terry RF, van der Rijt T. Overview of research activities associated with the World Health Organization: results of a survey covering 2006/07. *Health Research Policy and Systems*, 2010,8:25. doi: http://dx.doi.org/10.1186/1478-4505-8-25 PMID:20815938.
3. Decoster K, Appelmans A, Hill P. A health systems research mapping exercise in 26 low- and middle-income countries: narratives from health systems researchers, policy brokers and policy-makers. Geneva, World Health Organization, 2012.
4. UNDP/World Bank/WHO Special Programme for Research and Training in Tropical Diseases (TDR). Research capacity building in developing countries. Geneva, World Health Organization and TDR, 2003.
5. Planning, monitoring and evaluation framework for capacity strengthening in health research. (ESSENCE Good practice document series. Document TDR/ESSENCE/11.1). Geneva, World Health Organization, 2011.
6. Bates I et al. Indicators of sustainable capacity building for health research: analysis of four African case studies. *Health Research Policy and Systems*, 2011,9:14. doi: http://dx.doi.org/10.1186/1478-4505-9-14 PMID:21443780.
7. Capacity building in research. London, Department for International Development, 2010.
8. Fathalla MF, Fathalla MMF. A practical guide for health researchers. Cairo, World Health Organization Regional Office for the Eastern Mediterranean, 2004.
9. Gilson L, ed. Health policy and systems research: a methodological reader. Geneva, World Health Organization, 2012.
10. Ghaffar A et al. The 3D Combined Approach Matrix: an improved tool for setting priorities in research for health. Geneva, Global Forum for Health Research, 2009.
11. Okello D, Chongtrakul P, COHRED Working Group on Priority Setting. A manual for research priority setting using the ENHR strategy. Geneva, Council on Health Research for Development, 2000.
12. A manual for research priority setting using the essential national health research strategy. Geneva, Council on Health Research for Development, 2000.
13. Rudan I et al. Setting priorities in global child health research investments: universal challenges and conceptual framework. *Croatian Medical Journal*, 2008,49:307-317. doi: http://dx.doi.org/10.3325/cmj.2008.3.307 PMID:18581609.
14. Rudan I et al. Evidence-based priority setting for health care and research: tools to support policy in maternal, neonatal, and child health in Africa. *PLoS Medicine*, 2010,7:e1000308. doi: http://dx.doi.org/10.1371/journal.pmed.1000308 PMID:20644640.
15. Health technology assessment programme. London, National Institute for Health Research, 2013. (www.hta.ac.uk/funding/HTAremit.shtml, accessed 20 March 2013).

16. Policy research programme, best evidence for best policy. London, Department of Health, 2013. (prp.dh.gov.uk, accessed 20 March 2013).

17. Youngkong S, Kapiriri L, Baltussen R. Setting priorities for health interventions in developing countries: a review of empirical studies. *Tropical Medicine & International Health*, 2009,14:930-939. doi: http://dx.doi.org/10.1111/j.1365-3156.2009.02311.x PMID:19563479.

18. George A et al. Setting implementation research priorities to reduce preterm births and stillbirths at the community level. *PLoS Medicine*, 2011,8:e1000380. doi: http://dx.doi.org/10.1371/journal.pmed.1000380 PMID:21245907.

19. Lawn JE et al. Setting research priorities to reduce almost one million deaths from birth asphyxia by 2015. *PLoS Medicine*, 2011,8:e1000389. doi: http://dx.doi.org/10.1371/journal.pmed.1000389 PMID:21305038.

20. Rudan I et al. Setting research priorities to reduce global mortality from childhood pneumonia by 2015. *PLoS Medicine*, 2011,8:e1001099. doi: http://dx.doi.org/10.1371/journal.pmed.1001099 PMID:21980266.

21. Fontaine O et al. Setting research priorities to reduce global mortality from childhood diarrhoea by 2015. *PLoS Medicine*, 2009,6:e41. doi: http://dx.doi.org/10.1371/journal.pmed.1000041 PMID:19278292.

22. Tomlinson M et al. Setting priorities in child health research investments for South Africa. *PLoS Medicine*, 2007,4:e259. doi: http://dx.doi.org/10.1371/journal.pmed.0040259 PMID:17760497.

23. Sharan P et al. Mental health research priorities in low- and middle-income countries of Africa, Asia, Latin America and the Caribbean. *The British Journal of Psychiatry*, 2009,195:354-363. doi: http://dx.doi.org/10.1192/bjp.bp.108.050187 PMID:19794206.

24. Tol WA et al. Research priorities for mental health and psychosocial support in humanitarian settings. *PLoS Medicine*, 2011,8:e1001096. doi: http://dx.doi.org/10.1371/journal.pmed.1001096 PMID:21949644.

25. Nicolau I et al. Research questions and priorities for tuberculosis: a survey of published systematic reviews and meta-analyses. *PLoS ONE*, 2012,7:e42479. doi: http://dx.doi.org/10.1371/journal.pone.0042479 PMID:22848764.

26. An international roadmap for tuberculosis research: towards a world free of tuberculosis. Geneva, World Health Organization, 2011.

27. Lienhardt C et al. What research Is needed to stop TB? Introducing the TB research movement. *PLoS Medicine*, 2011,8:e1001135. doi: http://dx.doi.org/10.1371/journal.pmed.1001135 PMID:22140369.

28. Priorities in operational research to improve tuberculosis care and control. Geneva, World Health Organization, 2011.

29. The malERA Consultative Group on Drugs. A research agenda for malaria eradication: drugs. *PLoS Medicine*, 2011,8:e1000402. doi: http://dx.doi.org/10.1371/journal.pmed.1000402 PMID:21311580.

30. The malERA Consultative Group on Health Systems and Operational Research. A research agenda for malaria eradication: health systems and operational research. *PLoS Medicine*, 2011,8:e1000397. doi: http://dx.doi.org/10.1371/journal.pmed.1000397 PMID:21311588.

31. McDowell MA et al. Leishmaniasis: Middle East and North Africa research and development priorities. *PLoS Neglected Tropical Diseases*, 2011,5:e1219. doi: http://dx.doi.org/10.1371/journal.pntd.0001219 PMID:21814585.

32. Costa CH et al. Vaccines for the leishmaniases: proposals for a research agenda. *PLoS Neglected Tropical Diseases*, 2011,5:e943. doi: http://dx.doi.org/10.1371/journal.pntd.0000943 PMID:21468307.

33. Research priorities for Chagas disease, human African trypanosomiasis and leishmaniasis. Geneva, World Health Organization, 2012.

34. Dujardin JC et al. Research priorities for neglected infectious diseases in Latin America and the Caribbean region. *PLoS Neglected Tropical Diseases*, 2010,4:e780. doi: http://dx.doi.org/10.1371/journal.pntd.0000780 PMID:21049009.

35. Research priorities for helminth infections. Geneva: World Health Organization, 2012.

36. Research priorities for zoonoses and marginalized infections. Geneva, World Health Organization, 2012.

37. Prioritized research agenda for prevention and control of noncommunicable diseases. Geneva, World Health Organization, 2012.

38. Ranson MK et al. Priorities for research into human resources for health in low- and middle-income countries. *Bulletin of the World Health Organization*, 2010,88:435-443. doi: http://dx.doi.org/10.2471/BLT.09.066290 PMID:20539857.

39. Ranson K, Law TJ, Bennett S. Establishing health systems financing research priorities in developing countries using a participatory methodology. *Social Science & Medicine*, 2010,70:1933-1942. doi: http://dx.doi.org/10.1016/j.socscimed.2010.01.051 PMID:20378228.

40. Jones R, Lamont T, Haines A. Setting priorities for research and development in the NHS: a case study on the interface between primary and secondary care. *British Medical Journal*, 1995,311:1076-1080. doi: http://dx.doi.org/10.1136/bmj.311.7012.1076 PMID:7580669.

41. Östlin P et al. Priorities for research on equity and health: towards an equity-focused health research agenda. *PLoS Medicine*, 2011,8:e1001115. doi: http://dx.doi.org/10.1371/journal.pmed.1001115 PMID:22069378.

42. The 10/90 report on health research 1999. Geneva, Global Forum for Health Research, 1999.

43. Sizemore CF, Fauci AS. Transforming biomedical research to develop effective TB vaccines: the next ten years. *Tuberculosis (Edinburgh, Scotland)*, 2012,92:Suppl 1S2-S3. doi: http://dx.doi.org/10.1016/S1472-9792(12)70003-3 PMID:22441154.

44. Pacheco Santos LM et al. Fulfillment of the Brazilian agenda of priorities in health research. *Health Research Policy and Systems*, 2011,9:35. doi: http://dx.doi.org/10.1186/1478-4505-9-35 PMID:21884575.

45. Alger J et al. [National health research systems in Latin America: a 14-country review]. *Revista Panamericana de Salud Pública*, 2009,26:447-457. PMID:20107697.

46. Ijsselmuiden C, Ghannem H, Bouzouaia N. Développement du système de recherche en santé: analyse et établissement des priorités en Tunisie [Development of health research system: analysis and defining priorities in Tunsia]. *La Tunisie Medicale*, 2009,87:1-2. PMID:19522419.

47. Tomlinson M et al. A review of selected research priority setting processes at national level in low and middle income countries: towards fair and legitimate priority setting. *Health Research Policy and Systems*, 2011,9:19. doi: http://dx.doi.org/10.1186/1478-4505-9-19 PMID:21575144.

48. McKee M, Stuckler D, Basu S. Where there is no health research: what can be done to fill the global gaps in health research? *PLoS Medicine*, 2012,9:e1001209. doi: http://dx.doi.org/10.1371/journal.pmed.1001209 PMID:22545025.

49. The Paris Declaration on Aid Effectiveness and the Accra Agenda for Action. Paris, Organisation for Economic Co-operation and Development, 2005.

50. Fourth High Level Forum on Aid Effectiveness. Busan, Global Partnership for Effective Development Cooperation, 2011. (www.aideffectiveness.org/busanhlf4/, accessed 20 March 2013).

51. Kok MO et al. The emergence and current performance of a health research system: lessons from Guinea Bissau. *Health Research Policy and Systems*, 2012,10:5. doi: http://dx.doi.org/10.1186/1478-4505-10-5 PMID:22321566.

52. Lansang MA, Dennis R. Building capacity in health research in the developing world. *Bulletin of the World Health Organization*, 2004,82:764-770. PMID:15643798.

53. Bennett S et al. Building the field of health policy and systems research: an agenda for action. *PLoS Medicine*, 2011,8:e1001081. doi: http://dx.doi.org/10.1371/journal.pmed.1001081 PMID:21918641.

54. Hoffman SJ et al. A review of conceptual barriers and opportunities facing health systems research to inform a strategy from the World Health Organization. Geneva, World Health Organization, 2012.

55. Whitworth JA et al. Strengthening capacity for health research in Africa. *Lancet*, 2008,372:1590-1593. doi: http://dx.doi.org/10.1016/S0140-6736(08)61660-8 PMID:18984193.

56. Ijsselmuiden C et al. Africa's neglected area of human resources for health research – the way forward. South African Medical Journal/Suid-Afrikaanse tydskrif vir geneeskunde, 2012, 102:228–233.

57. How to build science capacity. *Nature*, 2012,490:331-334. doi: http://dx.doi.org/10.1038/490331a PMID:23075964.

58. Bennett S et al. What must be done to enhance capacity for health systems research? Geneva: World Health Organization2010.

59. Whitworth J, Sewankambo NK, Snewin VA. Improving implementation: building research capacity in maternal, neo-natal, and child health in Africa. *PLoS Medicine*, 2010,7:e1000299. doi: http://dx.doi.org/10.1371/journal.pmed.1000299 PMID:20625547.

60. Meyer AM, Davis M, Mays GP. Defining organizational capacity for public health services and systems research. *Journal of Public Health Management and Practice*, 2012,18:535-544. PMID:23023278.

61. Nwaka S et al. Developing ANDI: a novel approach to health product R&D in Africa. *PLoS Medicine*, 2010,7:e1000293. PMID:20613865 doi: http://dx.doi.org/10.1371/journal.pmed.1000293 PMID:20613865.

62. *The world health report 2006 – working together for health*. Geneva, World Health Organization, 2006.

63. Ijsselmuiden C. Human resources for health research. *MMS Bulletin*, 2007,104:22-27..

64. Guidelines for research in partnership with developing countries: 11 principles. Bern, Swiss Commission for Research Partnership with Developing Countries, (KFPE), 1998.

65. Kariuki T et al. Research and capacity building for control of neglected tropical diseases: the need for a different approach. *PLoS Neglected Tropical Diseases*, 2011,5:e1020. doi: http://dx.doi.org/10.1371/journal.pntd.0001020 PMID:21655352.

66. Garcia CR, Parodi AJ, Oliva G. Growing Latin American science. *Science*, 2012,338:1127. doi: http://dx.doi.org/10.1126/science.1232223 PMID:23197500.

67. Harries AD, Zachariah R. Applying DOTS principles for operational research capacity building. Public Health Action, 2012.

68. Laabes EP et al. How much longer will Africa have to depend on western nations for support of its capacity-building efforts for biomedical research? *Tropical Medicine & International Health*, 2011,16:258-262. doi: http://dx.doi.org/10.1111/j.1365-3156.2010.02709.x PMID:21371216.

69. *UK health research analysis 2009/10*. London, UK Clinical Research Collaboration, 2012.

70. Head MG et al. UK investments in global infectious disease research 1997–2010: a case study. *The Lancet Infectious Diseases*, 2013,13:55-64. doi: http://dx.doi.org/10.1016/S1473-3099(12)70261-X PMID:23140942.

71. Terry RF et al. Mapping global health research investments, time for new thinking - a Babel Fish for research data. *Health Research Policy and Systems*, 2012,10:28. doi: http://dx.doi.org/10.1186/1478-4505-10-28 PMID:22938160.

72. The Global Plan to Stop TB 2011–2015. Transforming the fight towards elimination of tuberculosis. Geneva, World Health Organization, 2010.

73. Tuberculosis Research and Development: 2011 report on tuberculosis research funding trends, 2005–2010. New York, NY, Treatment Action Group, 2012.

74. Zachariah R et al. The 2012 world health report 'no health without research': the endpoint needs to go beyond publication outputs. *Tropical Medicine & International Health*, 2012,17:1409-1411. doi: http://dx.doi.org/10.1111/j.1365-3156.2012.03072.x.

75. Lienhardt C, Cobelens FG. Operational research for improved tuberculosis control: the scope, the needs and the way forward. *The International Journal of Tuberculosis and Lung Disease*, 2011,15:6-13. PMID:21276290.

76. Five keys to improving research costing in low- and middle-income countries. (ESSENCE Good practice document series. Document TDR/ESSENCE/1.12). Geneva, World Health Organization, 2012.

77. Mahmood S et al. Strategies for capacity building for health research in Bangladesh: Role of core funding and a common monitoring and evaluation framework. *Health Research Policy and Systems*, 2011,9:31. doi: http://dx.doi.org/10.1186/1478-4505-9-31 PMID:21798006.

78. Nwaka S et al. Analysis of pan-African Centres of excellence in health innovation highlights opportunities and challenges for local innovation and financing in the continent. *BMC International Health and Human Rights*, 2012,12:11. doi: http://dx.doi.org/10.1186/1472-698X-12-11 PMID:22838941.

79. Lang TA et al. Clinical research in resource-limited settings: enhancing research capacity and working together to make trials less complicated. *PLoS Neglected Tropical Diseases*, 2010,4:e619. doi: http://dx.doi.org/10.1371/journal.pntd.0000619 PMID:20614013.

80. Mabey DC et al. Point-of-care tests to strengthen health systems and save newborn lives: the case of syphilis. *PLoS Medicine*, 2012,9:e1001233. doi: http://dx.doi.org/10.1371/journal.pmed.1001233 PMID:22719229.

81. Good research practice: principles and guidelines. London, Medical Research Council, 2012.

82. Australian Code for the Responsible Conduct of Research. Canberra, National Health and Medical Research Council, 2007.

83. The ethics of research related to healthcare in developing countries. London, Nuffield Council on Bioethics, 2005.

84. Singapore Statement on Research Integrity. Singapore, Second World Conference on Research Integrity, 2010.

85. Operational guidelines for ethics committees that review biomedical research. Geneva, World Health Organization, 2000.

86. UK Research Integrity Office (web site). Falmer, Sussex Innovation Centre, University of Sussex, 2012. (www.ukrio.org, accessed 20 March 2013).

87. WMA declaration of Helsinki. Ethical principles for medical research involving human subjects. Seoul, World Medical Association, 2008.

88. Standards and operational guidance for ethics review of health-related research with human participants. Geneva, World Health Organization, 2011.

89. Chalmers I, Haines A. Commentary: skilled forensic capacity needed to investigate allegations of research misconduct. *British Medical Journal*, 2011,342:d3977. doi: http://dx.doi.org/10.1136/bmj.d3977.

90. Chan M et al. Meeting the demand for results and accountability: a call for action on health data from eight global health agencies. *PLoS Medicine*, 2010,7:e1000223. doi: http://dx.doi.org/10.1371/journal.pmed.1000223 PMID:20126260.

91. Walport M, Brest P. Sharing research data to improve public health. *Lancet*, 2011,377:537-539. doi: http://dx.doi.org/10.1016/S0140-6736(10)62234-9 PMID:21216456.

92. The Royal Society. Science as an open enterprise: open data for open science. London, The Royal Society, 2012.

93. Rani M, Buckley BS. Systematic archiving and access to health research data: rationale, current status and way forward. *Bulletin of the World Health Organization*, 2012,90:932-939. PMID:23284199.

94. Leung E et al. Microcolony culture techniques for tuberculosis diagnosis: a systematic review. [i–iii.]. *The International Journal of Tuberculosis and Lung Disease*, 2012,16:16-23. doi: http://dx.doi.org/10.5588/ijtld.10.0065 PMID:21986554.

95. Haak LL et al. Standards and infrastructure for innovation and data exchange. *Science*, 2012,338:196-197. doi: http://dx.doi.org/10.1126/science.1221840 PMID:23066063.

96. International Clinical Trials Registry Platform (ICTRP) Geneva, World Health Organization, 2012. (www.who.int/ictrp/trial_reg/en/index2.html, accessed 20 March 2013).

97. World report on knowledge for better health – strengthening health systems. Geneva, World Health Organization, 2004.

98. Green A, Bennett S, eds. Sound choices: enhancing capacity for evidence-informed health policy. Geneva, World Health Organization, 2007.

99. Jamison DT et al. Disease control priorities in developing countries, 2nd ed. New York, NY, Oxford University Press, 2006.

100. Duflo E. Rigorous evaluation of human behavior. *Science*, 2012,336:1398. doi: http://dx.doi.org/10.1126/science.1224965 PMID:22700919.

101. Cobelens F et al. Research on implementation of interventions in tuberculosis control in low- and middle-income countries: a systematic review. *PLoS Medicine*, 2012,9:e1001358. doi: http://dx.doi.org/10.1371/journal.pmed.1001358 PMID:23271959.

102. Brooks A et al. Implementing new health interventions in developing countries: why do we lose a decade or more? *BioMed Central Public Health*, 2012,12:683. doi: http://dx.doi.org/10.1186/1471-2458-12-683 PMID:22908877.

103. Wasi P. "Triangle that moves the mountain" and health systems reform movement in Thailand. *Human Resources for Health Development Journal*, 2000,4:106-110..

104. Lavis JN et al. Assessing country-level efforts to link research to action. *Bulletin of the World Health Organization*, 2006,84:620-628. doi: http://dx.doi.org/10.2471/BLT.06.030312 PMID:16917649.

105. Glasgow RE, Emmons KM. How can we increase translation of research into practice? Types of evidence needed. *Annual Review of Public Health*, 2007,28:413-433. doi: http://dx.doi.org/10.1146/annurev.publhealth.28.021406.144145 PMID:17150029.

106. Panel on Return on Investment in Health Research. Making an impact: a preferred framework and indicators to measure returns on investment in health research. Ottawa, Canadian Academy of Health Sciences, 2009.

107. Orton L et al. The use of research evidence in public health decision making processes: systematic review. *PLoS ONE*, 2011,6:e21704. doi: http://dx.doi.org/10.1371/journal.pone.0021704 PMID:21818262.

108. Noonan RK, Emshoff G. Translating research to practice: putting "what works" to work. In: DiClemente RJ, Salazar LF, Crosby RA, eds. Health behavior theory for public health. Burlington, MA, Jones & Bartlett Learning, 2011:309–334.

109. Kok MO, Schuit AJ. Contribution mapping: a method for mapping the contribution of research to enhance its impact. *Health Research Policy and Systems*, 2012,10:21. doi: http://dx.doi.org/10.1186/1478-4505-10-21 PMID:22748169.

110. Boaz A, Baeza J, Fraser A. Effective implementation of research into practice: an overview of systematic reviews of the health literature. *BMC Research Notes*, 2011,4:212. doi: http://dx.doi.org/10.1186/1756-0500-4-212 PMID:21696585.

111. Dearing JW. Applying diffusion of innovation theory to intervention development. *Research on Social Work Practice*, 2009,19:503-518. doi: http://dx.doi.org/10.1177/1049731509335569 PMID:20976022.

112. Panisset U et al. Implementation research evidence uptake and use for policy-making. *Health Research Policy and Systems*, 2012,10:20. doi: http://dx.doi.org/10.1186/1478-4505-10-20 PMID:22748142.

113. Lavis JN et al. SUPPORT Tools for evidence-informed health Policymaking (STP). *Health Research Policy and Systems*, 2009,7:Suppl 1:I1. doi: http://dx.doi.org/10.1186/1478-4505-7-S1-I1 PMID:20018098.

114. Lewin S et al. Guidance for evidence-informed policies about health systems: assessing how much confidence to place in the research evidence. *PLoS Medicine*, 2012,9:e1001187. doi: http://dx.doi.org/10.1371/journal.pmed.1001187 PMID:22448147.

115. Bosch-Capblanch X et al. Guidance for evidence-informed policies about health systems: rationale for and challenges of guidance development. *PLoS Medicine*, 2012,9:e1001185. doi: http://dx.doi.org/10.1371/journal.pmed.1001185 PMID:22412356.

116. Buse K, Mays N, Walt G. Making health policy (Understanding public health), 2nd ed. New York, NY, Open University Press, 2012.

117. Strategy on health policy and systems research: changing mindsets. Geneva, World Health Organization, 2012.

118. Kebede M et al. Blueprints for informed policy decisions: a review of laws and policies requiring routine evaluation. Oslo, Kunnskapssenteret (Norwegian Knowledge Centre for the Health Services), 2012.

119. Giedion U, Alfonso EA, Díaz Y. The impact of universal coverage schemes in the developing world: a review of the existing evidence. Washington, DC, The World Bank, 2013.

120. Commission on Health Research for Development. Health research – essential link to equity in development. Oxford, Oxford University Press, 1990.

121. Research and development to meet health needs in developing countries: strengthening global financing and coordination. Report of the consultative expert working group on research and development: financing and coordination. Geneva, World Health Organization, 2012.

122. Research and development coordination and financing. Report of the Expert Working Group. Geneva, World Health Organization, 2010.

123. Knutsson KE et al. *Health policy/systems research, realizing the initiative – a background document to an international consultative meeting at Lejondal, Sweden April 10–12*. Lejondal, 1997 (unpublished).

124. Røttingen J-A et al. Mapping of available health research and development data: what's there, what's missing, and what role is there for a global observatory? *Lancet*, 2013, May 17. pii:S0140-6736(13)61046-6. doi: http://dx.doi.org/10.1016/S0140-6736(13)61046-6 PMID:23697824

125. Global strategy and plan of action on public health, innovation and intellectual property. Geneva, World Health Organization, 2011.

126. Hotez PJ et al. Strengthening mechanisms to prioritize, coordinate, finance, and execute R&D to meet health needs in developing countries. Washington, DC, Institute of Medicine, 2013.

127. Orphanet. The portal for rare diseases and orphan drugs (web site). Paris, Orphanet/INSERM, 2012 (www.orpha.net, accessed 20 March 2013).

128. Sow SO et al. Immunogenicity and safety of a meningococcal A conjugate vaccine in Africans. *The New England Journal of Medicine*, 2011,364:2293-2304. doi: http://dx.doi.org/10.1056/NEJMoa1003812 PMID:21675889.

129. Frasch CE, Preziosi MP, LaForce FM. Development of a group A meningococcal conjugate vaccine, MenAfriVac(TM). *Human Vaccines & Immunotherapeutics*, 2012,8:715-724. doi: http://dx.doi.org/10.4161/hv.19619 PMID:22495119.

130. Kennedy A et al. National health research system mapping in 10 Eastern Mediterranean countries. *Eastern Mediterranean Health Journal*, 2008,14:502-517. PMID:18720615.

131. National health research systems in Pacific island countries. Manila, World Health Organization Regional Office for the Western Pacific, 2009.

132. A new pathway for the regulation and governance of health research. London, Academy of Medical Sciences, 2011.

Action on research for
universal health coverage

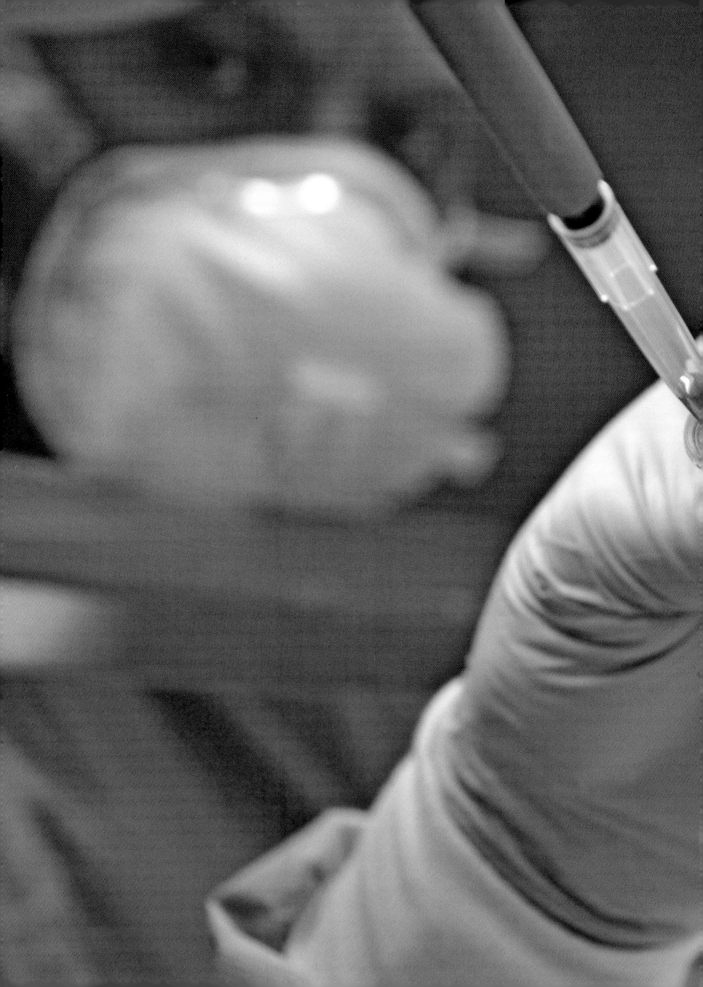

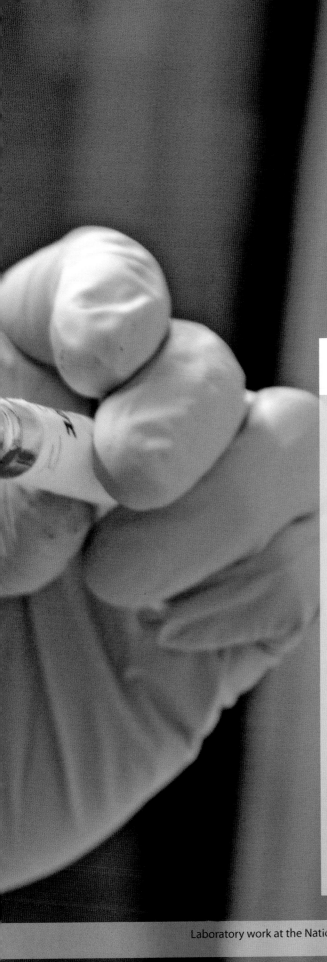

Chapter 5

Laboratory work at the National Institute of Epidemiologic Diagnosis and Reference (InDRE) Mexico City, Mexico (WHO/PAHO/Harold Ruiz).

Key points

Drawing on previous chapters, Chapter 5 highlights the dominant themes of the report, and proposes a set of actions to guide the conduct of research and to support research for universal health coverage.

There are a number of important considerations regarding the conduct of research with a focus on national health research systems. For instance:

- Research is not merely an essential tool for improving health services; it is also a source of inspiration for public health.

- While the research focus of this report is the improvement of access to health services and the protection of people at risk, the definition and measurement of progress towards universal health coverage are themselves topics for investigation.

- Wider coverage of health services and better financial protection usually lead to better health, but research is also needed to link the provision of services most effectively with health impact.

- Because local health problems often require local solutions, each country should be a producer as well as a consumer of research.

- Among the essential functions of national health research systems, developing human capacity is critical. The people who do the research are the foremost asset in the research enterprise and should be in the front line of capacity-strengthening.

- The long-observed gap between existing knowledge and health practice remains wide. Still greater effort is needed to translate evidence into policy and practice.

Actions to support research nationally and internationally include:

- monitoring (e.g. through the establishment of research observatories);

- coordination (from information-sharing to collaborative research studies);

- financing (to ensure that there are adequate funds to support global and local priorities in research).

WHO's role in carrying out and supporting research is articulated in the Organization's Strategy on Research for Health. The strategy aims to cultivate the highest quality research in order to deliver the greatest health benefits to the maximum number of people.

5

Action on research for universal health coverage

The goal of this report is not to measure definitively the gap between the present coverage of health services and universal coverage, but rather to identify the research questions that arise along the way to universal coverage and to discuss how these questions can be answered.

Chapter 1 identified two kinds of questions about research for universal health coverage. The first set of questions is about improving health and well-being – how to advance towards universal coverage, and how improved coverage protects and improves health. The second set of questions is about measurement – of the indicators that can be used as measures of the coverage of essential health services and financial risk protection in any setting.

In confronting these two sets of questions, the preceding four chapters have taken a broad view of research and a broad view of universal health coverage – where creativity and imagination are harnessed by the highest-quality science to deliver affordable health services and better health protection for everyone.

This final chapter highlights the dominant themes of the report and proposes a set of actions – first, on the conduct of research, with a focus on national health research systems and second, to support research nationally and internationally (Box 5.1). As part of the narrative, the chapter also outlines WHO's role in supporting these actions, based on the Organization's Strategy on Research for Health (Box 4.1) (*1*).

Research – essential for universal coverage and a source of inspiration for public health

The question "how can we reach universal health coverage?" almost always calls for a formal investigation of some kind, whether it be a randomized controlled trial or a simple observational study. On the road to universal coverage, taking a methodical approach to formulating and answering questions is not a luxury but a necessity; it is the source of objective evidence that can inform health policy and practice.

However, research is more than an essential tool; it is also a source of inspiration and motivation in public health. The discoveries made by research stir

Box 5.1. Principal questions and actions on research for universal health coverage

This box identifies the key questions about research for universal health coverage that arise from discussion in the main text, together with some important actions that can be taken to help answer the questions.

Questions on research

Improving the coverage of health services:

- How can essential health services and financial risk protection be made accessible to everyone? How do wider service coverage and better financial protection – and ultimately universal health coverage – lead to better health?

Measuring the coverage of health services:

- What indicators and data can be used to monitor progress towards universal coverage of essential health services and financial risk protection in each setting?

Actions on the conduct of research, mainly within national health research systems

Setting research priorities:

- Set priorities for research, especially at national level, on the basis of evaluations of the major causes of ill-health.

Strengthening research capacity:

- Give priority to recruiting, training and retaining the people who do research; research staff are the foremost asset of any research enterprise.
- Provide training not only in research methods but also in the good conduct of research – on accountability, ethics, integrity and the stewardship of information on behalf of others.
- Train policy-makers to use the evidence from research, and train researchers to understand the process of decision-making and health practitioners.

Setting standards:

- Refine and implement codes of practice to carry out ethical and responsible research in each setting.
- Classify types of research study and research data according to internationally agreed and comparable standards.

Translating research into policy and practice:

- Embed research within policy-making processes in order to facilitate the dialogue between science and practice.
- Establish formal procedures for translating evidence into practice.
- Ensure that programmes of continuing professional development, and for improving the quality of care, reflect the best available evidence.
- Enhance incentives to carry out research that is relevant to health policy.
- Engage private research companies along with public institutions in the discovery, development and delivery of new technologies.

Ensuring participation and public understanding of research:

- Include broad representation from society in the process of research governance.
- Increase public access to policy debates and evaluations both via the media and through public consultations and meetings.

Actions to support research, nationally and internationally

Monitoring research:

- Develop national and international research observatories to compile and analyse data on the process of doing research (funding, priorities, projects, etc.) and on the findings of research – including research aimed at achieving universal health coverage.

continues ...

... continued

Coordinating research and sharing information:

- Promote knowledge-sharing, network-building and collaboration, especially within and between countries that are beginning to develop research capacity.

Financing research:

- Develop improved mechanisms for raising and disbursing funds for research, either through existing national and international bodies or by creating new ones.
- Establish flexible funding mechanisms that permit research across disciplines, both within and beyond the health sector.
- Set criteria for investment in health research.

Managing and governing health research:

- Systematically evaluate management and governance in national and international health research systems, assessing whether mechanisms exist to carry out the essential functions above (on priorities, capacity, standards and translation).
- Systematically evaluate public policies and large-scale social programmes that are based on research for health, and make the results widely accessible.

ambitions to defeat the greatest public health problems, as two recent examples show. First, following the development of a new high-efficacy meningococcal A conjugate vaccine (MenAfriVac), 100 million people were vaccinated across the African meningitis belt within two years (*2, 3*). Second, the now-famous clinical trial HPTN 052 – *Science* magazine's "breakthrough of the year" for 2011 – showed how antiretroviral therapy can prevent almost all sexual transmission of HIV between couples, exciting further debate about eliminating HIV/AIDS (*4*).

None of the rising indicators of research activity described in Chapter 2 is, on its own, a guarantee of products and strategies that will help us reach universal health coverage. Collectively, however, these upward trends signal the growing volume of information and evidence that will influence health policy and practice in low- and middle-income countries. Most countries around the world now have, at least, the foundations on which to build effective national health research systems. Some have much more than the foundations; they have thriving research communities.

Defining and measuring progress towards universal health coverage

Because the causes of ill-health and the capacity for financial protection differ from one country to another, each nation must determine its own priority health problems, decide what services are needed to address these problems, and investigate how those services can be provided. The services that make up a national health system are usually too numerous to monitor comprehensively. The practical alternative is to choose a set of measurable coverage indicators to represent, as tracers, the overall quantity, quality and equitable delivery of the services to be provided, including ways to ensure financial protection. This leads to a pragmatic interpretation of universal coverage in any given setting so that each representative intervention, whether a health service or a mechanism of financial protection, is accessible to all who are eligible.

By definition, universal coverage guarantees access to services and financial protection for everyone. However, when coverage is partial, some people may benefit more than others. For this reason, measures of coverage should reveal, not simply the average accessibility of services in a population, but also the coverage among different groups of people classified by income, gender, ethnicity, geography and so on. Chapter 1 noted that the greatest progress in providing services for maternal and child health has been made by narrowing the gap between those with the lowest and those with the highest incomes (5). This is a form of "progressive universalism" in which the poorest individuals gain at least as much as the richest on the way to universal coverage (6). The point about measurement, however, is that disaggregated data must be applied to the right indicators in order to monitor the implementation of a chosen policy on equity.

From these considerations, two kinds of research questions arise. The first group of questions deals with improving health. Given the burden of disease in any setting, what services are needed, how can universal coverage of these services be achieved, and how does wider coverage lead to better health? This first group of questions is the principal concern of this report.

The second set of questions is about measurement: what is the practical definition of universal health coverage in any setting, and which indicators and data can be used to measure progress towards that goal? The answers will come partly from the large body of existing information on specific indicators, but new research will also be required. One product of this research will be a set of common indicators for comparing progress towards universal coverage across all countries.

It will often be possible to satisfy the definition of universal coverage with regard to one, several or perhaps all monitored health services – immunization against measles, access to antiretroviral therapy for people living with HIV infection, a particular type of health insurance, and so on.

But achieving this will inevitably prompt further questions about improving health, and the list of questions will grow as the changing causes of ill-health are tracked by new interventions and technologies. The response to previous successes and new challenges is to formulate a more ambitious definition of universal coverage – a new research agenda – and to generate yet more evidence to inform health policy and practice. Seeking universal health coverage is a powerful mechanism for continuing to seek better health.

The path to universal health coverage, and the path to better health

Chapter 3 presented 12 case-studies that showed, by example, how research can help to achieve universal health coverage and deliver results that actually, or potentially, influence health policy and health outcomes. There are many such examples that are not described in this report, but two from Chapter 3 that deal with service coverage and financing are revisited here. First, randomized controlled trials conducted in Ethiopia, Kenya, Sudan and Uganda showed that sodium stibogluconate (SSG) plus paromomycin (PM) are effective when used in combination to treat visceral leishmaniasis. The treatment can be shorter than with SSG alone and is less likely to generate drug resistance (7). On the basis of this evidence, WHO recommended that SSG and PM could be used as a first-line treatment for visceral leishmaniasis in East Africa. Second, a systematic review of evidence from Brazil, Colombia, Honduras, Malawi, Mexico and Nicaragua found that conditional cash transfers (CCTs) were associated with increased use of health services and better health outcomes (8). These findings will stimulate further research studies of the utility of CCTs in other countries.

As well as linking research to service coverage and then to health, the 12 case-studies also yield some general conclusions about doing research. Some of these concern the scope of research. The questions about how to achieve universal health coverage range from questions about the causes of ill-health, through methods for prevention and treatment, to questions about the performance of health services. Research must find out how to improve the coverage of current interventions and how to introduce new ones. Research must explore the development and use of both "software" (such as schemes for service provision) and "hardware" (R&D for commodities and technology). And research is needed to investigate ways of improving health from within and outside the health sector.

The case-studies also illustrate research methods, processes and outcomes. In general, successful research stimulates, and is stimulated by, a cycle of enquiry in which questions lead to answers that lead to yet more questions. The design of a research study is usually a compromise because the most robust evidence and the strongest inferences typically come from the most costly and lengthy studies (e.g. randomized controlled trials). The choice of design also depends on the need to generalize from one setting to another; results are more likely to be widely applicable when there are fewer and less variable processes linking causes and effects. Thus clinical trials tend to be favoured, for instance, to assess the efficacy of drugs and vaccines (governed by physiological factors), but observational studies are often used to resolve operational questions about how drugs and vaccines are best delivered by health services (influenced by local systems and behaviours). The unavoidable question facing every research study is "How much time and money can we afford to spend on the investigation?"

While this report has focused on research directed at achieving universal health coverage, it has also highlighted the co-benefits for health of research done in other sectors, such as

agriculture, education, environment and transport (Box 2.6). The report has not discussed research that will show how to make health systems more resilient to environmental threats such as extreme climate events, or research into how health systems can reduce their own greenhouse gas emissions. These are important subjects for research, but ancillary to the main theme of research for universal health coverage.

Research for universal health coverage in every country

As was made clear in Chapter 3, the results of some research studies are widely applicable but many of the steps towards universal health coverage will be made by finding local answers to local questions. For this reason, all nations need to be producers as well as consumers of research.

To become productive in research requires a functional national research system. Such a system must have the capacity to set priorities; to recruit staff and build research institutions; to adapt, adopt and maintain research standards; to use research to influence health policy and practice; and to monitor and report on the processes, the outputs, the outcomes and impact.

The priorities for research in each setting should be determined by the dominant health problems. Although curiosity-driven investigations have an essential place in the research landscape, this report places high value on studies that address major health concerns and which respond to present and future gaps in service coverage and financial risk protection. Standard methods have been devised to set research priorities, but the best-documented examples are those for specific health topics (Chapter 4). National exercises to set research priorities are less prominent, though some countries – notably Brazil – have taken a strong lead. To address the research priorities, once they have been chosen, investigations are needed throughout the research cycle: measuring the size of the health problem; understanding its cause(s); devising solutions; translating the evidence into policy, practice and products; and evaluating effectiveness after implementation.

The process of setting priorities should be inclusive, transparent, systematic, and linked to research funding. Those with a stake in the research process are diverse; they include decision-makers, implementers, civil society, funding agencies, pharmaceutical companies, product development partnerships, and researchers themselves. The roles of national and international research funding agencies – who have substantial leverage – include promoting high standards of objectivity, rigour and accountability, ensuring that the findings of results are made easily accessible, and demanding research accountability (namely that the funds available for research are used effectively).

Research for health has always been an international venture. The new trend is that long-established "north–south" links are being supplemented by "south–south" collaboration. The expertise of high-income countries will continue to be important because, for example, the burden of noncommunicable diseases, up to now largely a concern of the rich world, is growing in low-income countries. High-income countries also have a pool of trained researchers from low- and middle-income countries who, with the right incentives, may be encouraged to return home.

In a highly-connected world, the distinction between different kinds of international linkages is becoming less relevant. Connections of all sorts are needed to enhance peer-to-peer learning, to foster joint research endeavours, and to share resources. For nations that are emerging as forces in research, initiating a multinational collaboration, rather than simply joining as an invited participant, is a statement of growing research confidence.

Networking needs effective communication across the research community. Communication is easier in a common research language, which would require a uniform and systematic approach to the classification, collection and collation of data. Among systems for classifying types of research activity, a leading contender is the Health Research Classification System proposed by the European Science Foundation (9). Its purpose is to transmit the facts and findings of health research in a standard way to sponsors, governments and the public; to identify gaps and opportunities for research, which are vital in setting research priorities; to carry out comparable analyses of the quality and productivity of research output; to identify instances of research collaboration; and to streamline peer review and scientific recruitment.

Supporting the people who do research

Effective research requires transparent and accountable methods for allocating funds, and well-equipped research institutions and networks. However, it is the people who do research who are most critical to the success of the research enterprise. Consequently, the process of building research capacity should be spearheaded by staff recruitment and training, with mechanisms to retain the best researchers.

Research training is not only about learning scientific methods and techniques; it is also about the proper conduct of research. Codes of research ethics have been written to uphold honesty, objectivity, integrity, justice, accountability, intellectual property, professional courtesy and fairness, and good stewardship of research on behalf of others. The essential codes of practice are already in use in many countries. Although internationally agreed standards will often need to be updated and adjusted to local circumstances, an important future task is to implement the current standards in routine research practice everywhere.

Translating research evidence into health policy and practice

The important questions about health service coverage, and about health, need credible answers that are intelligible to those who can use them – i.e. decision-makers in various roles. When the findings of research are turned into policy and practice, a new set of questions arises for research.

Although a wide range of fundamental and applied research studies is essential to reach universal health coverage, the gap between existing knowledge and action is persistently large and is being closed only very slowly (*10*). Implementation and operational research, and health policy and systems research – bringing scientists and decision-makers together – are conspicuous areas of neglect.

To accelerate the process, research should be strengthened not only in academic centres but also in public health programmes that are close to the supply of, and demand for, health services. The greater the contact between researchers and policy-makers, the greater will be the mutual understanding. A variety of methods can be used to train decision-makers to use evidence from research, and to train researchers to understand the process of decision-making. The use of data (especially the large volume of data that are collected routinely), evidence and information can be illustrated in training courses to make clear the benefits of using evidence and the pitfalls of not doing so. Researchers may be employed in positions where they can help to frame policy-related questions which lend themselves to specific research studies, and to challenge decisions made about policy. Staff rotations between health ministries and research institutions are an aid to communication, and research staff employed explicitly to carry out knowledge translation will help to bridge the gap.

The application of research findings is more likely if there are formal procedures for translating evidence into practice. Mechanisms include the development of protocols for policy formulation, planning and implementation that explicitly refer to research evidence, and they include harnessing the skills of academics both in policy formulation and implementation. Publication is not the only, or even the best, measure of research productivity, but there are too few formal publications of routine operational research.

Translational research could be boosted with stronger incentives for the research community. To encourage a shared responsibility among researchers for reaching universal coverage, performance measures could be adjusted within academic and research institutions. Incentives should make reference, not only to publications in high-impact scientific and medical journals, but also to measures of influence on policy and practice.

In making the link between research and policy, private for-profit research companies (in areas such as biotechnology, pharmaceuticals, etc.) are just as important as public research organizations. A growing number of health products are being created through partnerships between the public and private sectors, making explicit links between various organizations involved in the discovery, development and delivery of new technologies. In this respect, Chapter 2 described the role of DNDi in coordinating the development of anthelmintic drugs by several pharmaceutical companies.

To fully exploit the results of research, scientists and decision-makers of all kinds need public support. It has been pointed out that civil society has a role in setting research priorities, but public engagement in research should be wider in scope. Members of the public, who are the source of government funds for research, are entitled to share in all aspects of the investigative process; their continued backing depends on being able to listen to, understand, believe in and make use of the results. Public engagement via the media, policy debates and open evaluations, works towards these ends. Making data publicly accessible (e.g. via the observatories described below) increases transparency and fosters greater public trust when evidence is used to make decisions that affect access to health care.

Just as a single research project does not necessarily generate a useful health product, a useful product does not necessarily influence health policy. This is because research is only one of the determinants of policy. Furthermore, the factors that influence health policy are not necessarily the same as those that help turn policy into practice (*11*, *12*). In addition to scientific evidence, other considerations are cultural values, human rights, equity and social justice, and competing demands for public spending (*13*, *14*). Because policy and practice are subject to various influences, and are decided in the face of multiple competing interests, robust and unbiased evidence ought to be valued by decision-makers.

Supporting research for universal health coverage, nationally and internationally

Chapter 4 discussed three mechanisms that support research for universal health coverage: monitoring, coordination and financing. Given the commitment to share data, a global observatory, linked to national observatories, could serve several functions in supporting research for universal health coverage more generally. A network of observatories could compile, analyse and present data on financial flows for health research, whether for technological development (traditional R&D) or for the improvement of health systems and services, and could link financing to research needs. Such a network could chart progress on research for universal health coverage by measuring each of the elements of the results chain, from inputs and processes, through outputs and outcomes, to health impact (Chapter 1). In practice, the number of tasks that could be carried out by observatories depends on the resources available and the will to develop them.

Monitoring by observatories, or a similar mechanism, also provides opportunities to coordinate research activities. Guidance on coordination could be provided by an international body, such as a reconstituted WHO Advisory Committee on Health Research (the first such advisory committee was established in 1956). Whichever body is responsible, it must represent the views of all concerned – researchers, funding agencies, private companies, and civil society and their representative governments in the countries concerned.

With regard to financing, international donors and national governments should measure their commitments to investing in health research against defined criteria. Chapter 4 listed some of the proposals that have been made – for instance, that "developing" countries should commit 0.05–0.1% of GDP to government-funded health research of all kinds (*15*). Some form of assessment is needed to judge whether investments are commensurate with achieving universal health coverage.

Once criteria have been chosen, mechanisms are needed for raising and disbursing funds, nationally and internationally. An improved system of financing might be newly created, or could be developed by existing organizations. Several international bodies – such as TDR, the GAVI Alliance, the Global Fund to Fight AIDS, Tuberculosis and Malaria and UNITAID – have the potential to manage research funds and distribute them for research in low- and middle-income countries.

Whatever funding mechanism is chosen, it should actively encourage research across disciplines, both within and beyond the health sector. As we have argued throughout this report, research for universal health coverage recognizes that health, and particularly prevention, depends on actions taken outside the health sector – in agriculture, education, employment, fiscal policy, social services, trade and so on. A comprehensive health policy must consider "heath in all sectors" of governance, and research must cover all these sectors too.

This will become still clearer when, from 2015 onwards, the world adopts a new development agenda to succeed the MDGs. In the post-2015 era, health must play a clearly articulated role in social, economic and human development (*16*). To generate evidence in support of sustainable development, funding must be available to underpin research for health across a range of disciplines. National and international committees that advise on health research must prepare for this new challenge.

WHO's role in research for universal health coverage

This report began with the observation that universal health coverage underpins "the attainment by all peoples of the highest possible level of health", which is a pillar of WHO's constitution and a guiding force in all the Organization's work. Throughout the report we have explained why research is vital for achieving universal health coverage, and consequently for improving the health of all people around the world.

The WHO Strategy on Research for Health (Box 4.1) is a mechanism to support health research whereby WHO works alongside governments, funding agencies, partnerships, non-governmental and civil society organizations, philanthropists and commercial investors, among others. Simply put, the goal of the WHO strategy is to cultivate the highest-quality research that delivers the greatest health benefits to the maximum number of people. In keeping with the essential functions needed to carry out research (Chapter 4 and above), WHO's role is to advance research that addresses the dominant health needs of its Member States, to support national health research systems, to set norms and standards for the proper conduct of research, and to accelerate the translation of research findings into health policy and practice.

As the principal international agency for health, WHO has a key role in promoting and conducting research for universal health coverage. In terms of monitoring, a global research observatory needs wide representation, should be able to develop and apply appropriate standards, and should garner the necessary international support. In terms of coordination, WHO hosts numerous research advisory committees with wide representation. And in terms of financing, TDR and UNITAID, both hosted by WHO, are potential mechanisms for disbursing research funds. As these possibilities are explored further, WHO is working to reinforce core functions. One of these is to ensure that the Organization's own guidelines reflect the best available evidence from research.

References

1. *WHO strategy on research for health*. Geneva, World Health Organization, 2012. (http://www.who.int/phi/WHO_Strategy_on_research_for_health.pdf, accessed 23 April 2013).

2. Sow SO et al. Immunogenicity and safety of a meningococcal A conjugate vaccine in Africans. *The New England Journal of Medicine*, 2011,364:2293-2304. doi: http://dx.doi.org/10.1056/NEJMoa1003812 PMID:21675889

3. Frasch CE, Preziosi MP, LaForce FM. Development of a group A meningococcal conjugate vaccine, MenAfriVac(TM). *Human Vaccines & Immunotherapeutics*, 2012,8:715-724. doi: http://dx.doi.org/10.4161/hv.19619 PMID:22495119

4. Cohen MS et al. Prevention of HIV-1 infection with early antiretroviral therapy. *The New England Journal of Medicine*, 2011,365:493-505. doi: http://dx.doi.org/10.1056/NEJMoa1105243 PMID:21767103

5. Victora CG et al. How changes in coverage affect equity in maternal and child health interventions in 35 Countdown to 2015 countries: an analysis of national surveys. *Lancet*, 2012,380:1149-1156. doi: http://dx.doi.org/10.1016/S0140-6736(12)61427-5 PMID:22999433

6. Gwatkin DR, Ergo A. Universal health coverage: friend or foe of health equity? *Lancet*, 2011,377:2160-2161. doi: http://dx.doi.org/10.1016/S0140-6736(10)62058-2 PMID:21084113

7. Musa A et al. Sodium stibogluconate (SSG) & paromomycin combination compared to SSG for visceral leishmaniasis in East Africa: a randomised controlled trial. *PLoS neglected tropical diseases*, 2012,6:e1674. doi: http://dx.doi.org/10.1371/journal.pntd.0001674 PMID:22724029

8. Lagarde M, Haines A, Palmer N. The impact of conditional cash transfers on health outcomes and use of health services in low and middle income countries. *Cochrane database of systematic reviews (Online)*, 2009,4:CD008137. PMID:19821444

9. *Health research classification systems: current approaches and future recommendations*. Strasbourg, European Science Foundation, 2011.

10. *World report on knowledge for better health – strengthening health systems*. Geneva, World Health Organization, 2004.

11. Grol R, Grimshaw J. From best evidence to best practice: effective implementation of change in patients' care. *Lancet*, 2003,362:1225-1230. doi: http://dx.doi.org/10.1016/S0140-6736(03)14546-1 PMID:14568747

12. Bosch-Capblanch X et al. Guidance for evidence-informed policies about health systems: rationale for and challenges of guidance development. *PLoS Medicine*, 2012,9:e1001185. doi: http://dx.doi.org/10.1371/journal.pmed.1001185 PMID:22412356

13. National Center for Science and Engineering Statistics. *Science and engineering indicators 2012*. Arlington, VA, National Science Foundation, 2012.

14. Humphreys K, Piot P. Scientific evidence alone is not sufficient basis for health policy. *BMJ (Clinical research ed)*, 2012,344:e1316. doi: http://dx.doi.org/10.1136/bmj.e1316 PMID:22371864

15. *Research and development to meet health needs in developing countries: strengthening global financing and coordination. Report of the Consultative Expert Working Group on Research and Development: Financing and Coordination*. Geneva, World Health Organization, 2012.

16. *Sustainable development goals*. New York, NY, United Nations, 2013. (sustainabledevelopment.un.org, accessed 20 March 2013).

Index

Note: Pages suffixed by b, f, or t refer to boxes, figures or tables respectively.